Fight Autism and Win

Biomedical Therapies That Actually Work!

Second Edition

By:

Jan Martin, Tressie Taylor

Unraveled Publishing

Fight Autism and Win: Biomedical Therapies That Actually Work!

Second Edition

Copyright © Jan Martin, Tressie Taylor

Cover Design: Jan Martin

Publishing Date: July 2013, March 2012

ISBN 10 digit: 0-615-85154-1

IBSN 13 digit: 978-0-615-85154-9

Publisher Name:

Unraveled Publishing
1749 E. Lawn, Unit V
Springfield, MO 65804
United States of America

Foreword

This book really was a labor of love. In the early days, finding solid information on recovering our children meant hours of searching various books, websites, and forums. It is a daunting task to sort out the real, helpful information from the latest fads which only empty our wallets and waste precious time. Through personal experience, as well as years of helping parents, we have been able to sort through the rhetoric and learn the most effective therapies. Once we'd developed a more effective way of recovering our children, we wanted to share it with parents in an organized and straightforward way. Eventually our first book was born. The feedback we received from parents was truly inspiring. It is very rewarding to know that our years of hard work have been such a benefit for so many families. This book is our most recent endeavor which contains updated information so that we can continue to reach more parents. When we read posts from parents describing their child's progress it warms our hearts making all the struggles and hard work worthwhile. So from our hearts to yours, we share how we put our children on the road to recovery!

We want to thank all the parents who trusted us, listened to us, and supported us along the way. We also want to thank Dr. Andrew Hall Cutler, for his research, his books, and his ongoing participation in public forums. His willingness to share his time and knowledge is a blessing to us all (Thank you Andy). Your work has helped us get our children and our lives back.

Best in Recovery,

Jan Martin

Tressie Taylor

Table of Contents

Stories of Healing and Hope

Yun: 3 year old daughter, 50 rounds: "My daughter regressed directly after the MMR shot at 20 months old and was diagnosed at 2 ½ years old. Two weeks after the diagnosis, we started sugar-free, gluten-free, casein-free and soy-free diet. Two months later we began AC chelation. Now she is 3.10 years old, and we have done 50 rounds of AC chelation and 2 rounds of high dose vitamin A protocol.

I was afraid to do the ATEC test when we started; it would have been too devastating to know she was so severe and low functioning. In retrospect I would say her ATEC number would have been around 120 when things were the worst. After 8 to 10 rounds of chelation, I did the first ATEC test and she scored 95. Now after 50 rounds her score is 40. Her physical health has made the most improvements. Cognitive and receptive language is improving with the rounds too. Her cognition and expressive language is still very limited for her age and I know we still have a long way to go. But tonight is a peaceful night because I know she is really improving."

Sarah: 4 year old son, 17 rounds: "This book is the most direct and informative book I've read on an autism intervention and I have read a lot of books! For a parent who is exhausted, doesn't have any free time, and is desperate for something to help their child, a brief and concise book is a blessing. The chapters are also set up to make it a valuable resource to come back to over and over again.

We finally found Andy Cutler's protocol after a year of mistakenly thinking we had to clean up my son's gut before approaching his heavy metal toxicity. Looking back, it's hard to know that we wasted all that time. We also tried high-dose chelation suppositories which unfortunately caused scary side effects. Along with the side effects came some great gains though, so we knew chelation was needed, but in a safer way. Low frequent dose chelation has been a life changer for our family.

From FAW, I first figured out that my son had many symptoms of adrenal fatigue. This had never come up in a year and a half of seeing a DAN doctor regularly. Within days of adrenal glandular supplementation, my son's quality of life dramatically improved. His blood sugar leveled out which eliminated his mood crashes and "drug addict" carb cravings. His overall and unpredictable emotional roller coaster completely disappeared.

His moments of jumping back and forth between laughing and crying went away and never came back. After adjusting the dosage his sleep greatly improved. He used to sleep through the night about twice a month. Now he wakes up at night less than once a week. After adjusting the dosage a bit more, we were able to decrease the discomfort and cranky feelings he had at the end of his chelation rounds.

Other than removing dairy and gluten from his diet, adrenal support was my son's biggest miracle worker until AC chelation started.

When we started the low frequent dose protocol we were seeing incredible gains by the second round. He was more observant of the world around him, putting together larger processes in his day, tolerating new situations for the first time, naturally staying "with" us out in public, using eye contact to check in with us and read our faces, and much more. By round three everyone in his life had cried happy tears for one reason or another. His therapists, teachers, and family members were all reporting fantastic gains even without being aware that we had started chelation. I didn't tell anyone we started something new yet still the positive reports started pouring in!

We are now 17 rounds in and I can't even describe all the changes without writing a book. So many people in our life make comments about how any certain situation used to cause him stress, or would cause us stress trying to deal with him! And now so many things in our life are breathtakingly easier. He feels better, he is more confident, more aware, more engaged, more well rested, and just doing great in general.

I wrote a blog post around round 10 because we were overjoyed with how amazing our new life felt! (And we still are)

We just can't wait to see how he's doing after a few years of chelation! Finding this protocol and having the FAW Yahoo group as a priceless resource for getting questions answered has lifted a huge burden from our shoulders. I used to think and hope that maybe my son had a chance at recovery but now I KNOW he has a chance at recovery. We are thrilled and relieved and so thankful for the parents who have gone before us and laid the path for us to follow. Because of the book and the email group I knew exactly what to buy, where to get it, how and when to administer the doses, and how to trouble shoot. I couldn't ask for anything else!"

Deepa: 16 year old son, 135 rounds: "My boy was 13 when I first heard about AC chelation. In those 13 years we had tried various things, some seemed to help a little, some did nothing. The more I read about this protocol, the science of it stuck with me. The hair test met the counting rules and my first thought was "those metals have no business being in my child's body; they need to be cleaned out". I knew we were dealing with an older child, so how much damage could be reversed was a huge question. But with the continued support from FAW I was confident to start chelation and kept at it through various setbacks.

The book contains everything that was shared in the online forum and some more. It's like a ready reference when I have a question. I have learned to read my non-verbal child better, differentiate between yeast, bacteria and parasite and adrenal issues and address them effectively. We have not seen any wows but I do feel that he has made progress in various areas. He is more responsive, less fidgety, willing to communicate, sleeps better. This is the place I have found the most sound and effective advice that has helped me all the way. My boy is 16 now; we have done 135+ rounds. We still have a very long way to go, but we have come a long way too. I wish I had known about this protocol earlier."

Fani: 18 year old son, 73 rounds: "Frequent-low-dose chelation protocol has given our son his life back! In addition to autism, he had so many health problems that just getting through the day without him being sick was something we desperately looked forward to. We started chelation when he was a young teen and are not done yet, but he now goes to college and his future looks bright!"

Haven: 13 year old son, 108 rounds: "We spent years doing diet and biomed. Our son's immune system was destroyed by vaccines. After his regression he suffered constant infections. He got an infection (sometimes multiple infections such as strep and staphylococcus at the same time) roughly every two weeks post-regression. It seemed that as soon as he was over one infection, we would get three or four good days, and here would come the next infection. He missed about fifty percent of the school year in the early years. This went on from 2001 -2010.

Some things got better with biomed and diet: speech, behavior, sleep, OCD (until IV chelation), stimming (until IV). The progress was slow though I realize he did better than many others in regaining reciprocal and functional expressive speech.

The problem was nothing mainstream doctors or DAN physicians suggested did anything to improve his immune function. All they did was label him with "Immune Disorder NOS." Our lives revolved around sickness, and my son had to miss out on a lot of things because if we planned something he would inevitably come down with a fever and then we couldn't do whatever it was we planned.

His trips to the emergency room and tier one medications they prescribed pretty much ruined us financially. It's hard to go from comfortable to worrying paycheck to paycheck about how to pay for things. The DAN docs didn't help much with this because no matter how much we told them "Do not order anything insurance won't pay for because we can't afford it" we would get big bills in the mail. Then we were talked into IV chelation and that was a disaster. My son had horrible reactions and once it triggered a severe asthma attack which then snowballed into pneumonia. My son has had pneumonia eight times since regression.

I had heard about AC very early on but was afraid to do it for many reasons that seem silly to me now. We finally began AC in January of 2011. It did not take long to notice improvements in asthma, reciprocal speech, focus, less anxiety, improvement in academic performance and most of all a significant improvement in immune function. Since we began AC our lives have not revolved around sickness all the time. He can hit a rough patch every now and then but overall his immune function has greatly improved and we are thrilled about it. Many members of our extended family have daily conversations with my son now and I love being able to talk to him. He still has a ways to go with speech and social skills but he is really catching up in academic areas. Since beginning AC, the future began to look a lot brighter."

Alison: 4 year old son, 75 rounds: "We have done around 75 rounds of AC protocol. In my opinion we have progressed from moderate autism to near recovery. He responded from round one. He started speaking more and began speaking in his second language. He had a lot of fears and phobias, limited speech, gross motor, fine motor issues. These are disappearing gradually with AC chelation. He's in preschool and has a couple of friends now whereas before he was very fearful of other children. We are now working on pragmatic speech. We still have remaining issues but I can see the light at the end of the tunnel! We started when my son was just 3, he is now 4 ½ now. We are currently doing anti-virals listed in the Fight Autism and Win book and we have noticed more awareness in all areas. This book makes it a lot easier for the parent to implement this protocol. I'm so happy my son is getting better. Thanks so much to Andy and the authors of this book"

Carrie: 7 year old son, 6 rounds: We began AC chelation in March 2013. I was beyond petrified to begin this on my son without the help of a doctor. I'd never taken my son's health into my own hands. We'd never seen a DAN doctor so I was 100% brand new to this.

Within about 4 rounds our son began making comments about how he'd miss his assistant teacher at school post-graduation. By round 5 after adding in ALA, his handwriting had improved. He had normal, detailed conversations with his older sister without any side effects. We'd never had this happen before. He began asking questions about things on TV and noticing little things around the house, etc. His improvements are very subtle but noticeable. It's as if he's able to put things together in his mind more easily than before

I think the supplement that has helped him most has been phosphatidylserine. He struggles with moodiness quite a bit. Starting the

GF/CF diet has kept him out of trouble at school. His teacher even noted how much better he is while on the diet.

Finding the FAW book/forum has been one of the best things that have happened in our lives. I can't imagine continuing down the road to more ADHD drugs. We've had adverse reactions to those and have been bounced around from one drug to another for years now. Seeing improvements this early leaves us hopeful that we'll get to drop meds for good one day!

Chapter 1
Autism Unraveled

Autism is a topic on every one's mind today as its prevalence continues to rise every year. Autism Spectrum Disorder (ASD) plagues millions of children worldwide and parents are left with few options and even fewer answers. It doesn't have to be this way. There are answers, there is hope.

We have heard the chanting of mainstream medicine, insisting that autism is genetic. They say autism is an inherited developmental disorder, psychological in nature, and therefore is essentially out of our control. We are told that the only possible treatments for our beautiful babies are psychotropic medications (mostly untested in children) and years and years of intensive and costly behavioral therapies. Not only that, but they doom our children to this lifelong impairment based solely and completely on a set of behaviors.

They ignore the physical symptoms of gut and digestive issues, autoimmune dysfunction, sensory disturbances, endocrine malfunction, increased prevalence of allergies, sleeping disorders, and worst of all physical pain. When parents bring these valid physical concerns to the attention of doctors they are often brushed aside.

One mother tells of her child with chronic constipation. She was told it was only behavioral, yet when she treated it with anti-fungals and probiotics her son's stools normalized and his pain went away.

Another mother tells us that her child never slept. Both he and his mother were chronically sleep deprived. Their ABA therapist had been trying to control this with behavioral intervention months without success. Yet, two weeks after endocrine support was started her son began sleeping through the night.

Then we have yet another story of a young child who never made eye contact, never initiated any kind of conversation, or social interaction. Only three days after her mother removed dairy from her diet she looks straight into her mother's eyes and says, "Come play with me."

While these stories are powerful, what is perhaps the most enlightening of all are the thousands of mercury toxic hair tests we've seen from children with autism. What is even more extraordinary is the fact that many of these children start talking for the first time when you begin to remove metals from their bodies.

In recent years there has been a lot of talk about mercury's role in autism and other developmental disorders. The reason for this concern is due to the increase in mercury exposure for children and its effects on the immune system and brain. You may be surprised to know that this is not the first time in history this set of developmental, behavioral, and physical disorders has been encountered in epidemic proportions.

One tragic example was Minimata disease, which is described as a neurological disorder characterized by peripheral sensory loss, tremors, ataxia and both hearing and vision loss. The cause was traced to the mercury contamination of Minamata Bay which led to the poisoning of more than 10,000 people.

Another well known instance of mercury poisoning was in Pink's disease. Infants suffered from symptoms like weepy red rash, peeling skin, lethargy, respiratory distress and general ill health. Children who were walking prior to contracting Pink Disease were reported to regress and lose this skill. In 1947 the cause was discovered to be mercury laden teething powders. After they were banned in 1950 the occurrence of Pink's became rare. A support group of adults who suffered from Pink's as infants also report increased prevalence of autoimmune conditions, chemical sensitivities, allergies, co-ordination difficulties, and a susceptibility to emotional and psychiatric disorders.

Mercury is one of the most toxic naturally occurring substances we are exposed too. Unfortunately the repercussions of these exposures to the health and development of children are often overlooked. Children are especially susceptible to damage from mercury because their exposures occur during the development of the brain.

It is not for us, however, to debate the many entities who define a certain set of behaviors as autism or who make claims about its cause. We are here only to report what we know works. We will leave you to look over the chart below and determine for yourself what your child's truth is. On the left you will find symptoms commonly associated with ASD. On the right you will see symptoms listed in medical textbooks as being observed in mercury toxicity.

Just remember mercury poisoning is curable!

Comparison of Characteristics of Autism and Mercury Poisoning[1]		
	Autism	Mercury Poisoning
Movement Disorders	Arm flapping, jumping, spinning, rocking, circling; abnormal posture and gait; clumsiness, uncoordinated; difficulties crawling, laying down, sitting, walking; difficulty swallowing or chewing; walking on the toes.	Arm flapping, ankle jerks, rocking, circling; uncoordinated, clumsiness; inability to walk, stand, or sit; difficulty swallowing or chewing; walking on toes.
Sensory Problems	Oversensitive to sound; abnormal sensation in the mouth, arms, and legs; doesn't like to be touched.	Oversensitive to sound; abnormal sensations in the mouth, arms, and legs; doesn't like to be touched.

[1] Cave MD, Stephanie. *What Your Doctor May Not Tell You About Children's Vaccinations.* Grand Central Publishing Sept. 2001. 63-64. Print

Speech, Hearing Problems	Delayed language or failure of speech to develop.	Mild to severe hearing loss; problems with speech.
Language Problems	Problems with articulation; word use errors.	Problems with articulation; word retrieval problems.
Cognitive Problems	Borderline intelligence; mental retardation: may be reversed; poor concentration, shifting attention; difficulty following multiple commands; difficulty comprehending words; difficulty understanding abstract ideas and symbols.	Borderline intelligence; mental retardation: may be reversed; poor concentration and attention; difficulty following complex commands; difficulty comprehending words; difficulty understanding abstract ideas and symbols.
Visual Problems	Poor eye contact; blurred vision.	Poor eye contact; blurred vision.
Physical Problems	Decreased muscle strength, especially in upper body, incontinence; rash, dermatitis; abnormal sweating, poor circulation, high heart rate; diarrhea, constipation, gas, abdominal pain; anorexia, feeding problems; seizures; tendency for allergies, asthma; family history of autoimmune symptoms like rheumatoid arthritis.	Decreased muscle strength, especially in upper body, incontinence; salivating; rash, dermatitis; abnormal sweating, poor circulation, high heart rate; abdominal pain; anorexia, nausea, poor appetite; seizures; sensitive individuals more likely to have allergies, asthma; more likely to have autoimmune symptoms, especially rheumatoid arthritis.

Unusual Behaviors	Sleeping difficulties; injures self, such as head banging; staring, unprovoked crying, and social isolation.	Sleeping difficulties; injures self, such as head banging; staring, unprovoked crying, and social isolation.

We have seen many therapies come and go over the years. Through our experiences with our own families as well as advising parents we have determined the most helpful therapies available. We put them at your fingertips so that your child can realize the same successes we have experienced. These therapies are simple and can be done by any parent. Your child can feel better and can achieve a greater level of health, which in turn, leads to improvement in function, behavior, and development.

There are many fad therapies out there today that are marketed to parents. Many of them are expensive or even dangerous and can make your child very uncomfortable. It is an absolute tragedy that so many parents spend their entire life savings on therapies that don't work or lead to regressions that are sometimes permanent. Over the years we have met thousands of parents online who report this very same story over and over again.

They went to Dr. so and so, who ran tons of tests, put their child on loads of supplements, they did this or that and $40,000 later, they have nothing to show for it in terms of any permanent improvements in their child. It is truly heartbreaking to hear their stories because it didn't have to happen.

There is another way. Children have been recovering with the methods in this book since the late 1990's. You won't find it in most medical literature or doctor's offices. You don't hear about it from the developmental pediatrician. Quite frankly it's not very profitable, because you can do this, yourself, at home. Your child doesn't need tons of follow-up appointments, prescription drugs, or frequent laboratory work. It is gentle, safe, and effective.

In the past the biggest challenge with this therapy has been simply finding it. If you are a parent with a newly diagnosed child this isn't in the diagnosis packet. Parents are in the throes of emotion and pain when they learn what their child is facing and they are at the mercy of mainstream information about autism. We don't want you to get lost in the sea of autism jargon. Just relax, make yourself a cup of tea, and curl up in your favorite chair for a good read. You can finally breathe knowing you have the solution at your fingertips.

Chapter 2

Heavy Metal Everywhere

Mercury, lead and other toxic metals can have a great impact on health and development. This is one of the biggest reasons parents continue to question what role they might play in Autism. So many of our children test positive for metals and have a-positive response to chelation. So many of our children are mercury toxic, but how did they get that way?

Mercury is everywhere and it is a cumulative poison. When children are continually exposed to mercury, it accumulates in their body and begins to have a negative impact on their health. This is referred to as the "toxic tipping point". It is the point at which health and development become significantly impaired. The time this takes varies from person to person because some people can get rid of mercury much more quickly than others. Each child has an individual toxic tipping point that will be affected by how much mercury they are exposed too and how sensitive they are to it.

Many of us are not aware of the many sources of mercury in our environment. Mercury pollution is the result of a growing number of industrial applications. It is used in compact fluorescent light bulbs (CFL's), light up tennis shoes, the production of high fructose corn syrup and more. Mercury is used in dental amalgams, some vaccines, mercury thermometers, blood pressure cuffs, and many other medical applications. Mercury is also a by-product of coal fired power plants emitting tons of coal ash per year. In the past it was found in Mercurochrome antiseptic, contact lens cleaning solutions, and glass thermometers, some of which may still be in use today. Unfortunately mercury is often disposed of improperly. We could stop at pointing our fingers at big industry dumping toxins into our water supply, but it can be even more insidious than that. For example, perhaps the previous tenants in your apartment broke a few CFL light bulbs on your living room or bedroom carpet. Maybe the children who lived in your house before you bought it were playing with the mercury from a broken thermometer and dropped it in your back yard. Because of things like this today mercury is in our soil, the air we breathe, the water we drink, and the homes we live in. It's virtually everywhere!

The good news is that, while you cannot control all the toxins your family is exposed too, you can avoid many sources of mercury by knowing where to look. For example: Pregnant women (and their growing babies) are often exposed through high mercury fish in their diets, dental work, and vaccines. Since these sources can be avoided a mother can reduce her infant's prenatal mercury exposure.

Fish are a common source of mercury throughout the world but are often a staple in many diets. This is especially problematic for pregnant women, women of child bearing age, and children. It is best to exclude all high mercury fish from your diet and if you do eat fish, chose only low mercury fish on occasion. In some cases when there seems to be a reaction to eating fish, such as vomiting, nausea or feeling ill, it is best to avoid it entirely during the chelation process.

Metal dental fillings, also called "silver" or amalgam fillings are another avoidable source of mercury. Amalgams are 49% mercury and continually emit mercury vapor into your body. The American Dental Association (ADA) holds the position that amalgams are safe, however, research has shown they do release mercury vapor and are one of the adult populations' largest sources of exposure.[2] You should insist on composite fillings for yourself and your family. If you have amalgams, avoid having dental work done while pregnant. Mercury amalgams must be removed safely before beginning chelation.[3]

---

[2] Koral DMD, Stephen M. *"The Case against Amalgam"*. International Academy of Oral Medicine and Toxicology: 2002, 2005. Web. 11 Nov. 2011.
<http://www.iaomt.org/articles/category_view.asp?intReleaseID=288&catid=30 2002, 2005>

[3] Koral DMD, Stephen M. *"Safe Removal of Amalgam Fillings"*. International Academy of Oral Medicine and Toxicology: 2002, 2007. Web. 11 Nov. 2011
<http://www.iaomt.org/articles/category_view.asp?intReleaseID=288&catid=30 >

Vaccines are another source that must be considered. Pregnant women are encouraged to receive the flu vaccine, but it is one of the vaccines in which thimerosal (a mercury containing preservative) has not been removed. Even vaccines that do not contain mercury are problematic in pregnancy by exposing the fetus to aluminum, formaldehyde, and a host of other toxic chemicals. It is important to avoid all mercury containing vaccinations. Many parents are being assured that the newer "thimerosal-free" vaccines are safer but they have their own set of problems. These vaccines are not completely free of mercury. They now contain only trace amounts, which makes the term "thimerosal-free" misleading. In fact, while the total amount of mercury has been reduced, large amounts of aluminum have been added in its place. Mercury and aluminum are synergistic metals[4] which may make these vaccines just as toxic as the original full thimerosal versions. Further complicating the vaccine issue is that many doctors continue to give children the cheaper, mercury preserved vaccines that are sold for adults only. After all, they've been told a million times vaccines are perfectly safe!

We cannot ignore the growing number of parental reports of ASD children regressing after receiving vaccinations. Others report a continual worsening of their child following each round of vaccines. Parents should be informed about these reports so that they know that there are risks involved in vaccination. It is important that during the chelation process vaccine exposure to metals is strictly avoided. Continued exposure to new mercury sources like vaccines or amalgams would not be safe during the chelation process. This can cause serious problems and prevent recovery.

Many parents are not familiar with the vaccine laws, but, in most states and countries, exemption forms are available even for the "mandatory" vaccines. Parents often file philosophical or religious exemptions. Medical exemptions are also an option for children who have had a reaction to vaccines or are medically fragile. You can file the appropriate papers to avoid vaccines and

---

[4] Synergistic metals: interaction of two or more metals such that the total effect is greater than the sum of the individual effects

still be in compliance with laws for school. There are many websites and support forums that can assist you with this information if you need it.

A key part of recovering your child from metal poisoning and ensuring their future health is to try to avoid or reduce all controllable sources of mercury and heavy metals, including lead, aluminum, antimony, silver[5] etc.

---

[5] Colloidal silver is often used medicinally but is problematic for individuals with mercury toxicity and should be avoided.

Chapter 3
Testing Toxicity

Testing for heavy metals can be done fairly easily using a couple of truly effective methods. Many practitioners do use other tests but these seem to be ineffective or only measure the previous few days of exposure. Much of these testing methods originate with the diagnosis of acute environmental exposure in the work place, not chronic lower level exposures as seen in autism.

Hair Elements Testing specifically from Doctors Data Inc., is a basic, inexpensive, and non-invasive way of looking for heavy metals. This is the preferred method of heavy metal testing. It will show what metals your body has excreted over the past three months, as well as various minerals. While mercury can show up as significantly elevated on the test, it is more common for it to hide, showing little to no mercury excretion. This sometimes leads practitioners to believe mercury isn't a problem. In order to interpret these tests correctly you have to look for the effect mercury has on the essential minerals. Mercury interferes with how minerals are handled in the body and causes something referred to as "deranged mineral transport". Therefore, it is important to use the proper method to interpret your child's hair tests. Dr. Andrew Hall Cutler, PhD has worked extensively with these tests to establish a reliable method for interpretation. This involves looking at the arrangement of the essential minerals, as well as the toxic metals. This method is referred to as the "counting rules"[6]. This test can also be a helpful indicator of adrenal function, thyroid function, and malabsorption issues.

---

[6] Cutler PhD, PE, Andrew Hall. *Hair Test Interpretations: Finding Hidden Toxicities. First Ed.* Washington: Andrew Hall Cutler, PhD, PE, 2004. 16-26.. Print

We highly recommend you buy *"Hair Test Interpretation: Finding Hidden Toxicities"* by Andrew Hall Cutler PhD[7] so that you can interpret this test effectively on our own.

It is important to note that supplements can influence the results and sometimes make a test look better than it would have otherwise. Therefore a test that does not meet rules may still be toxic by other factors especially if there was known mercury exposure.

Tracking Symptoms and Past Exposures is a very effective means of gauging whether or not metals may be a problem, especially when testing is not available or inconclusive.

- Does your child suffer medical problems that doctors cannot cure, but offer only symptoms control?

- Did your child's health change following a vaccine or dental work?

- Has your child suffered developmental delays, regressions or a loss of skills?

- Did you have any dental work done during pregnancy?

- Was your child vaccinated?

- Did/does your child have metal dental fillings? Do you?

- Are you chemically sensitive (MCS)?

- Do you suffer from any "syndrome", allergies, chronic fatigue, digestive ailments, fibromyalgia etc?

---

[7] Cutler PhD, PE, Andrew Hall. *Hair Test Interpretations: Finding Hidden Toxicities. First Ed.* Washington: Andrew Hall Cutler, PhD, PE, 2004. Print.
<http://www.noamalgam.com/hairtestbook.html>

- Has your child been diagnosed with a developmental disorder?

This is just a basic list of things that may indicate your child has been exposed to heavy metals and that they might be causing health or developmental problems for your child. If the hair test was inconclusive but there are any indications your child may have heavy metal toxicity consider doing 5-10 weekly rounds of chelation. If you see any changes in behavior either good or bad it is highly likely your child will benefit from chelation.

We will also mention some methods used by doctors so you are familiar with them. The following tests are not recommended and may be risky or ineffective.

Blood Testing is popular among main stream medical professionals. Blood tests are very accurate at diagnosing recent exposure which occurred in the past few days. This test was originally developed to diagnose acute high level exposure in the work place. The problem is that just because heavy metals clear the blood doesn't mean they clear the body. If your child is suffering from past exposure the metals have settled into bones, body tissues, and the brain. These metals are undetectable through blood testing.

Challenge Testing is a provoked urine test. We do not recommend these tests because they use one time, high doses of chelator. The idea is to "provoke" the excretion of metals, and then measure how much is excreted in the urine or feces. One issue with this test is that because metals exist in our environment, anyone given a chelator will show metals on excretion. This does not necessarily mean they are toxic. The second problem is that giving high doses of chelator in this manner causes damage by redistributing mercury into the brain. While this test can tell you metals are present in the body, it cannot tell you how much. Since mercury doesn't readily leave the brain and the chelators used in these tests do not cross the blood brain barrier, this test cannot measure brain mercury. There are safer ways to determine metal toxicity, so there is no reason to put your child at risk with high doses of chelators. Many people who have done this testing report terrible side effects or regressions. They have documented their experiences at www.dmpsbackfire.com where they describe what happened to them

13

when they were given infrequent, high doses of chelators similar to what is given for a "challenge test".

French Urine Porphyrins Testing is a medically recognized way to confirm mercury. Elevated porphyrins (proteins) occur when there are metals in the body causing blood cells to spill porphyrins into the urine. There are specific porphyrins that are spilled for mercury and specific ones for lead. This test must be done correctly and the specimen handled carefully because it is a very sensitive test. If it is not kept in the right conditions this test may be falsely negative and therefore may not be worth the investment.

Testing for metals can be managed easily using a non-invasive hair test or considering past exposures and a trial of chelation. There is no need to invest in costly blood work, urine testing or risky challenge testing.

Chapter 4
Half Life is Key

The human body has no natural mechanism to remove mercury from the brain. Once there, it is trapped and must be removed through other means. You can make its effects far worse by improper removal techniques like using chlorella, cilantro, EDTA, homeopathic chelation, etc., or by following improper chelation protocols like high dose intravenous (IV), the DMSA 10 mg per pound/8 hour protocol, or giving the chelators every other day etc. It is very important to understand the various chelation protocols out there and learn how to remove metals safely. Currently there is only one method that does this, frequent low dose chelation or as some parents fondly refers to it "Andy Cutler chelation".

This method was developed by Andrew Hall Cutler PhD, who began researching safer therapy to address his own mercury toxicity. Most of the chelation protocols in use had terrible side effects and increased problems by causing mercury to settle in the brain repeatedly. This made the patient become sicker over time. This process is known as "redistribution". Dr. Cutler developed a method to reduce the redistribution of mercury. He accomplished this by applying a basic chemistry principle known as pharmacokinetics or "half-life"[8]. This principle is based on how long a substance lasts in the body. Many medications are dosed by their half-life, which provides a steady blood level of the medicine over a period of time. This is the principle used to determine the dose and timing of many drugs currently in use. This is why certain antibiotics are dosed three times per day, or why pain medicine is generally given every four hours.

---

[8] DiPrio, Joseph T., William J. Spruill, William E. Wade, and Et Al. *Concepts in Clinical Pharmacokinetics*. Fifth ed. ASHP, 2010. Print.

By applying the rules of half-life to the chelators, you can minimize redistribution and avoid many of the symptoms that happen when chelators are taken randomly. This helps safely remove metals without causing serious side effects or risking further damage.

So how do chelators work? When chelators are given they "pull" metals by attaching to them, and clearing them from the body. The chelators have a two pronged effect, or claw by which they grab and hold onto the metal. They do not hold on tight but rather continuously drop and pick up metals until they eventually exit the body through-urine or feces. As long as there is a steady blood level of chelator this process will continue. When the levels of chelator in the blood drop and there is no longer anything to "grab" the dropped metals, they will be reabsorbed back into body tissue or what is called "redistributed".

This is a problem because mercury has a high affinity for fatty tissue, like the liver, thyroid, and brain and it is more likely that it will redistribute to these organs first. This means it is essential to reduce redistribution as much as possible during chelation.

There are numerous protocols on the Internet and in use by physicians that are said to remove heavy metals. Some of them are not safe, or worse, quite dangerous. This is not the case when frequent low dose chelation is done properly by sticking to the dosing and timing guidelines. On this protocol high doses are never given and intravenous medications are never used.

With frequent low dose chelation side effects are extremely minimal and controlled or eliminated by following the protocol and using supportive supplements. Should any significant symptoms occur on a round, you can adjust supplements, or stop the round and lower the chelator dose to reduce or eliminate symptoms for upcoming rounds.

Chapter 5
The Basic Four and More

There are four essential supplements you need to give your child while chelating. You should have your child on these four supplements for two weeks prior to chelation. These supplements help their bodies work better despite having mercury poisoning. They also reduce any of the side effects of chelation, such as fatigue. Supplements must be taken consistently on and off rounds. These supplements do not necessarily produce any gains in terms of autism symptoms but they do help maintain health.

Children need the following four essential supplements[9]:

- Magnesium: 300-600 mg per day divided into four doses.

- Vitamin C: 500-1000 mg per day divided into four doses

- Vitamin E: 400 IU per day (d-alpha tocopherol, not dl-alpha tocopherol). Vitamin E is a fat soluble supplement and those can be given once or more per day.

- Zinc: 1 mg per pound of weight + 20 mg divided into two or more doses per day. (Do not exceed 100 mg of zinc per day)

We also recommend a good quality multivitamin/mineral product if your child will tolerate it. There are other supplements which are recommended, but **not required** that do help improve how your child feels and functions (remember to subtract the amount in your multi).

---

[9] For children who weigh 100 pounds or more see Amalgam Illness by Dr Andrew Hall Cutler for adult dosages.

<u>Milk Thistle:</u> ¼-1 capsule (20-80 mg) 3-4 times per day, milk thistle as 80% silymarin. This is helpful for children who have bile issues, liver problems, constipation, brain fog or fatigue after a round. Anyone with chemical sensitivity, a sign of a sluggish liver, may benefit from this. Avoid if allergic to daisies.

<u>Vitamin A:</u> 5-10,000 IU per day including any cod liver oil (CLO). Do not count beta carotene towards the requirement because beta carotene is not efficiently converted into vitamin A by many children.

<u>B complex:</u> The equivalent of a B complex (12-25 mg) per day divided into three doses. It is advised to use yeast-free B supplements. A few kids may display hyperactivity with B vitamins given later in the day. Some children may not tolerate B's initially. You may need to chelate for 5-10 rounds and try them again. When giving B12 watch for irritability, hyperactivity or aggressions as these are common signs of intolerance.

<u>Vitamin D3:</u> 1-2,000 IU per day to maintain healthy levels. Since it supports immune health giving extra D in the winter can help prevent flu. Children with tooth decay usually need more vitamin D, calcium, and vitamin K. Children with hypothyroid issues should have their vitamin D level tested to rule out deficiency. If vitamin D levels are low up to 5,000 IU per day is helpful until this is corrected.

<u>Calcium:</u> 5-20 mg per pound, divided into 2-3 doses per day. This is very helpful for children who have lead poisoning, are dairy-free, or eat very limited sources of calcium. Hypothyroid children also have problems retaining and using calcium.

<u>Chromium:</u> 200 mcg daily. Children who display hypoglycemic symptoms such as irritability when it's close to meal time may need 100 mcg with every meal.

<u>Vitamin K:</u> 500-1000 mcg per day of K1 or K2 (preferable). K is needed to keep calcium where it belongs. Probiotics in our gut produce vitamin K but yeast overgrowth crowds out these good bacteria leaving many of our children deficient in K.

Molybdenum: 5-20 mcg per pound divided 2-3 doses over the day. It is especially useful with children high in copper if used with zinc. Children with lead poisoning should not use higher doses.

Selenium: 1-2 mcg per pound total divided into three doses over the day. Selenomethionine is the preferred form. Avoid selenium from yeast.

Adrenal Cortex Extract: This glandular is used for children who have symptoms of adrenal fatigue. Please refer to Chapter 12 to see if your child may need this.

Essential Fatty Acid (EFA): 1-3 tbsp per day. Use good quality fish oils that do not contain heavy metals or PCB's. Flax, borage, evening primrose and coconut oils are also sources of EFAs.

Lecithin: 1500-9000 mg, can improve memory and learning capacity. It is good for liver and/or ammonia issues, digestion, and helps the absorption of fat soluble vitamins like A, D, E, and cod liver oil. Phosphatidylcholine is a readily absorbed lecithin. Most supplements are made from soy; you may need to look for sunflower lecithin if you have an allergy to soy.

Remember these are optional and based on tolerance and needs of your child. Supplements dosed by weight apply to children up to 100 pounds.

Chapter 6

Chelation 101

There are two chelators which are used most often and are available for over the counter use in the U.S. These are DMSA (dimercaptosuccinic acid) and Alpha Lipoic Acid (ALA). ALA is also referred to as lipoic acid, not to be confused with alpha linolenic acid which is one of the beneficial fatty acids and is not a chelator.

You can begin chelation with either DMSA or ALA or a combination of DMSA/ALA. The only contraindications are related to recent mercury exposure from vaccines, amalgams or high fish consumption. If you have been exposed in the past three months you will need to wait three months to use ALA but you can begin DMSA as soon as 4 days after the exposure.

ALA (Alpha Lipoic Acid) is a water and fat soluble chelator that does cross the blood brain barrier and is the only chelator that can remove mercury and arsenic from the central nervous system and brain. ALA does not effectively remove lead or some other metals. If your only issue is mercury ALA is the only chelator needed. ALA is an antioxidant which regenerates glutathione (helps-detoxification) and supports liver function. Chelating with ALA only can increase adrenal symptoms in some and can cause spaciness. If this happens adding DMSA along with the ALA usually solves the issue.

DMSA is a water soluble chelator that removes mercury and other metals from the body only; it does not have the ability to cross the blood brain barrier. It is an effective chelator of lead and other metals and can increase excretion of mercury by up to 30% over ALA alone.

Most parents choose to begin with DMSA adding ALA somewhere between round 2 and 10. It's important to know that ALA is the main chelator and the only chelator that is able to remove mercury from the brain. ALA when used alone can sometimes cause foggy or spacey behavior.

It is also worth mentioning another chelator called DMPS (2, 3-dimercapto-1-propanesulfonic acid) which removes mercury from the body but not the brain. It can be beneficial when children do not do well on ALA alone and cannot use DMSA for some reason. In the US it is only available through a doctor.

The dosage for frequent-low-dose chelation is based on your child's weight. While the range is between $\frac{1}{8}$ mg-$\frac{1}{2}$ mg per pound, it is best to start at $\frac{1}{8}$ mg per pound. With children you should not exceed $\frac{1}{2}$ mg per pound.

DMSA is dosed by its half life of four hours around the clock, day and night, for the duration of the three day round. ALA is dosed by its half life of three hours during the day, with the option to dose at four hours at night, but only during the parent's sleep cycle. This means there are only two 4 hour stretches per 24 hours for the duration of the three day round. When using both DMSA/ALA, dose both chelators according to the schedule for ALA.

Late Dosing Guidelines: If a dose is more than 1 hour late redistribution has begun. Do not give the dose. You have to stop the round. You can begin again at the next scheduled round (usually next weekend). For DMSA/ALA or ALA only rounds on 4 hour night doses, you cannot dose any later than 30 minutes past the scheduled dose time. If the dose is missed by more than 30 minutes, end the round.

Early Dosing Guidelines: You can give a dose earlier if needed, but not later. For example dosing at 2.5 hours is acceptable. If a dose is given earlier adjust the next dose accordingly so that you are never dosing your child later than the maximum (4 hours for DMSA alone/3 hours for ALA or ALA+DMSA).

> Note: It is important to keep dosing times as steady as possible so, while dosing 30 min or so early once in awhile is fine, do not dose at 1 hour this time, then 3 hours, then 1.5 hours, then 2.5 hours, and so on.

A round is generally 72 hours. The minimum round length is 64 hours for those whose children are in school. You would start chelation the moment the child comes home from school on Friday and continue until the moment they leave for school Monday morning. Rounds less than 64 hours should be avoided due to a higher probability of unwanted side effects and more significant redistribution.

The minimum time between rounds is equal or greater to the time your child chelated. For most this is three days on and four days off, or one round per week (usually every weekend). You can chelate your child every other week, but this will double the overall time it takes to complete the recovery process so it is only recommended when absolutely necessary.

Generally you will see positive changes in your child within 5-10 rounds, but any change good or bad means the chelators are moving metals. It is helpful to keep a video journal and/or written diary of your child's symptoms, improvements, doses, round numbers etc. Follow up testing is not generally needed. Some parents do yearly follow up hair testing if they wish, but it is not required.

Sometimes chelation can cause a slight flare up in your child's symptoms. This usually wears off a day or two after the round has ended. In many children yeast flare ups will happen during chelation but they are easily controlled with probiotics and natural over-the-counter anti-fungals. Mild side effects like these are easily managed with the supplements that are discussed in detail in this book. Children are generally very comfortable and don't experience negative symptoms with this protocol.

The overall length of the chelation process varies based on your child's level of toxicity. Most will need between 100-300 rounds in order to complete the chelation process. The main point to remember is to stick to the dosing and timing guidelines. The key to recovery is to stay the course and not get discouraged at how long it may take. After all, the mercury didn't get in there over night; it's going to take time to get it out safely!

Chapter 7

Measure, Mix, and Dose

It will make things easier to buy the lowest dose capsules of the chelators you can find (usually 5-50 mg). When your child reaches higher doses you can purchase 100 mg capsules.

Measuring the doses: Calculate the dose your child needs using $\frac{1}{8}$ mg per pound as your starting point. Then divide that into the milligrams of the capsules you purchased to determine how many times you must divide the capsule contents to reach your child's desired dose.

Example:

50 pound child: $50 \div 8 = 6.25$

25 mg capsule: $25 \div 6.25 = 4$

Each 25 mg capsule will make four doses.

Suggested methods for dividing the powder:

- Empty the capsule onto a plate and divide the pile of powder equally using a knife/credit card…etc. Put those little piles into empty capsules, paper cups, shot glasses, etc., until they are to be given. Get the piles as equal as you can visually.

- Empty one 25 mg capsule of ALA into five tsp of liquid so that each chelator dose taken from the liquid would be a $\frac{1}{2}$ teaspoon or 5 mg. You can easily adjust the amount of liquid or ALA as your child's dosage changes. ALA can be premixed and stored for up to

24 hours. We do not recommend doing this with DMSA because of issues with oxidation.[10]

- Divide the chelator directly into empty capsules. For example: If you need 5 mg, take five small empty capsules and pour equal amounts of the 25 mg chelator into each, then put the caps back on. You can give the capsules if your child can swallow them, or open them as needed and mix them into food or drink. It can help to have a capsule machine to hold the empties for you.

Methods for administering the doses:

- Medicine Syringe (squirt)

- Medicine cup/teaspoon

- Mix it into food like applesauce, pudding or yogurt

- Mix into any juice or rice milk

- Teaching them to swallow tiny capsules

Other Useful Information:

- If your child has to take ALA in food or drink, rather than a capsule, provide a drink of water to wash it down because it is irritating to the mouth and throat.

- Premixed ALA will smell and taste stronger than freshly mixed. We do not recommend premixing DMSA.

---

[10] DMSA is not stable when mixed into liquid and will oxidize and loose potency. Previous recommendations have been that DMSA may be mixed into 'sufficiently tart' liquid and stored for 'up to' 12 hours, however, the rate of oxidation has not shown to be consistent.

- Cold liquids mask the taste better than warm ones.

- DMSA tastes like sulphur, smells like sulphur. Children do not seem to be bothered by this.

- Night dosing may be difficult at first but within a few rounds most children no longer wake up at all.

- Giving a small amount of antifungals with some of the chelator doses can help children who get yeast flares on rounds.

Ideas that we have used successfully:

"We are currently doing 12.5 mg of ALA only. I empty one 100 mg ALA cap into a baby food jar and add 8 teaspoons of orange juice. Mix well and store in fridge. For every dose I shake well and use a medicine syringe to give 1 tsp of the mix with a drink of water to wash it down. Works well day or night." — Tressie

"We use miniature peanut butter cups and cut them in half with a knife. Use a ¼ tsp measuring spoon to remove some of the peanut butter filling. Place that peanut butter into a small glass dessert cup, then add the chelator and mix the powder into the peanut butter. Spread the peanut butter back into the hollow peanut butter cup and put the lid back on. Give the child the peanut butter cup and follow it with a drink of water. You can also sprinkle some vitamin C or other supplements in with the chelator if desired." -Jan

Chapter 8
The Ebb and Flow

Some normal symptoms can occur during chelation. As metals are removed you may see a slight increase in some of the behaviors that the heavy metals were causing. It is also common to see symptoms or behaviors return that had previously disappeared. These usually last a short time before disappearing permanently. In other children, some behaviors leave, then return, then leave again. This may even happen several times before they are finally gone for good. These fluctuations in symptoms and behaviors are expected but can be easily managed by adjusting supplements. The following are some typical symptoms seen during chelation:

- Hyperactivity

- Fatigue

- Slight increase in urination/bed-wetting (temporary)

- Stimming

- Irritability

- Yeast

- Reduced appetite

- Increase in appetite

- Stool changes

- Sulfur smelling urine or stool

- Passing gas (flatulence)

- Low-grade fevers of 99°F can be seen in the first five rounds, but this is rare.

- Vivid dreams

- Difficulty falling or staying asleep (see Chapter 12)

If the symptoms are more than mildly uncomfortable, the chelator dose may be too high. In this case there are two options:

1. End the current round early and then begin with a lower dose at the next scheduled round. Do note that redistribution symptoms will be worse if you end early.

2. Finish the round at the current dose and increase antioxidant supplements and then lower the dose for the next round.

Do not adjust the chelator dose mid-round!

Common symptoms like fatigue or irritability improve by increasing vitamin C or magnesium. Epsom salt baths are also very helpful, particularly in children who may be hyperactive when chelating. Digestive symptoms during chelation are usually caused by yeast and would be helped by probiotics and anti-fungals.

During the early part of chelation a small number of children will experience an increase in urination which can result in bed wetting. Don't worry. It is temporary and usually subsides within the first 3-10 rounds. If a child is having trouble with bed wetting you might consider using diapers or pull-ups until this resolves itself.

Another symptom some children experience in the beginning of chelation is slightly elevated body temperatures of under 100 degrees Fahrenheit They may feel warm to the touch, or have red cheeks, but they are still eating, drinking, sleeping and playing normally. This isn't anything to worry about and usually goes away somewhere between rounds 3-10.

It is sometimes necessary to end a round early. Symptoms that signal a need to stop a round are as follows:

- Fever over 101 Fahrenheit

- Vomiting from illness/flu

- Extreme fatigue or lethargy

- A missed dose

The most common causes of vomiting, fever, and lethargy are colds and flu. When your child is ill, postpone chelation until they are well. This allows the body to focus on healing. Use your best judgment to determine whether or not your child is ill and should not chelate.

Fast Metabolizers:

If your child seems to become irritable, agitated or complains of a headache shortly before their next dose is scheduled, they may be a fast metabolizer. What this means is their metabolism processes the chelator quicker than other children. If you see these symptoms, even when on relatively low doses of chelator with proper support supplements in place, you should consider dosing the chelators sooner than three hours. You can try dosing every 2 ½ hours instead, to see if this resolves these symptoms. There are rare children who have extremely fast metabolisms and they may need 2 hour dosing. Keep in mind that this is not common. There is no benefit in dosing early unless your child has this issue. If you dose children with normal metabolisms too frequently it may increase yeast or adrenal symptoms.

Special Circumstances: Children who have seizure disorders require further consideration. Due to mercury and vaccination, many children with autism will develop seizures, at some point, if not properly chelated. Chelation itself does not cause seizures, but may aggravate an underlying or unknown seizure condition. If your child has seizures, or has one on a round, chelation should be postponed until an EEG (electroencephalogram) and evaluation can be done by a neurologist to determine if there is abnormal electrical activity. It is most useful to get a 24 hour EEG, because you seldom actually catch a seizure on the 1 hour test. You should get a copy of the interpretive report. Sometimes parents are told that the test was normal, or that it was "typical for a child with autism," but in fact, there was abnormal electrical activity found. Children do not always have obvious seizures during the test but abnormal readings may be present. If your child has an abnormal EEG, medication should be used to control the seizure activity and prevent any brain injury, then you can continue to chelate. Removing mercury is what will lead to ending seizures so lifelong medication isn't needed.

If your child begins to get frequent colds or infections it might be a good idea to test for low absolute neutrophils. A CBC (complete blood count) with differential will give you this measurement. Do not confuse total neutrophils with absolute neutrophils (ANC). The only measurement that you look at for this condition is the absolute neutrophil count. If your child's ANC results are below normal do not chelate with DMSA more than one round per month. DMSA can contribute to low neutrophil levels.

There are supplements which can help address low neutrophils and provide support until their levels return to normal. Children with this condition should have their ANC levels tested periodically to make sure they return to normal and do not fall too low. These children can chelate with ALA only or ALA only with occasional DMSA/ALA rounds.

It is important to remember that seizures and low neutrophils are rare problems, but they can be managed effectively in order to chelate and ultimately correct the problems.

Chapter 9
Raising the Dose: Stalling

Some of the most common questions most parents have are when and how to adjust chelator doses. They key is to remember that the optimum chelator dose is the one which produces improvements with as few side effects as possible. You might consider a dose increase if your child has completed at least five rounds at your current dose without any results, either positive or negative. The exception is with yeast symptoms which may not go away for many rounds.

If your child is doing well and you are not seeing symptoms then a reasonable dose increase would be done in 5 mg increments. For example if your child is on 5 mg of DMSA/ALA you would first increase to 10 mg of DMSA and maintain 5 mg of ALA the next round. If they tolerate the increase of the first chelator, you would then increase the ALA to 10 mg on the subsequent round. Then hold those doses for at least five more rounds.

It's good to remember that there is no need to raise your child's current dose if you still see improvements. You also shouldn't raise the chelators if there are moderate side effects on rounds, like irritability or stimming, which resolve between rounds.

It's important to know that the process of chelation won't move faster by trying to raise doses quickly to reach ½ mg per pound. What generally happens when rushing to raise doses is that you get an increase in yeast and significant adrenal stress. This leads to needing more breaks in chelation and ultimately slows the process down. Not to mention it is more uncomfortable for your child. Many children chelate successfully at low doses and may not need to reach ½ mg per pound.

If your child has any problems with a dosage increase, drop back to the previous chelator dose at the next round. You want your child to be comfortable with as few side effects as possible.

The Dreaded Stall: After you have chelated your child for some time they may experience something often referred to as "stall period" or a lack of progress. This happens to everyone and is actually part of the process.

Parents become discouraged when they hit this slump we call "stall" in progress especially if they don't expect it or know what's going on. Some will think it isn't working anymore, but it is. There is an expected path with chelation where you see improvements your first 3-7 months but then suddenly it may seem like nothing is happening. That's the stall. It can last from 4-15 months in some cases but typically it's about four months. And some parents report this happening more than once in their chelation journey.

So why does this happen? Well, when chelators are first introduced into the body they clear the blood of metals. This is where the metals are having the greatest impact on health and behavior.

As this metal burden decreases, your child will feel and function much better. Once enough metals have been removed from the blood, the body then begins to release them from the organs.

When the body dumps metals back into the blood, you will no longer see the kinds of gains that were apparent earlier. You may even see slight regressions although never back to their pre-chelation status. As long as you continue to chelate, the gains will return and your child will continue to improve as the total metal burden is reduced.

Think of the stall like spring cleaning. You straighten up, dust and vacuum the main rooms and your house looks nice but you've been "stashing" things in that closet by the door for awhile now. When you begin to clean that closet the living room will look temporarily worse. Once you get that closet nice and organized you will have to go back and re-clean your living room again.

You will have to keep cleaning and messing things up until all that stashed clutter is gone and your entire home is nice and organized. This is what happens with the stall period. It might seem like nothing good is happening, but it really is and eventually gains will start again. Most parents report stall periods between 3-6 months. This is why it's important not to get discouraged and stop! If you keep going you'll get all those cluttered closets cleaned out. It may take between 100-300 rounds to finish chelation depending on how toxic your child is, but once you have chelation underway you can work on other issues while you work through rounds. You can use stall periods to work on things like viruses, bacteria, or parasites while continuing chelation.

If you push through the stall period and continue to follow the protocols and manage symptoms as they come up, in no time your child will be on the path to healing and better health.

Chapter 10
Dental Matters

Since mercury amalgams (metal dental fillings) are a primary daily source of mercury exposure they need to be removed safely prior to beginning chelation. These fillings are black, silver or gray in appearance. This should be done by a properly trained dentist so you can chelate your child effectively. Many people have become more mercury poisoned by having their fillings drilled away without precautions to protect them from inhaled mercury. The International Academy of Oral Medicine and Toxicology has a safe protocol for removal available online at www.IAOMT.org.

Any amalgams should be replaced with composite fillings (white). It is important to be certain there isn't any amalgam under crowns or caps prior to chelation. You can verify this by removing the cap (crown) unless your child's dentist has the records and knows for certain that no amalgam was used or left in the crowned tooth. This also applies to root canals or pulp caps. Porcelain crowns are safe for chelation, provided there is no amalgam underneath them.

Composite (white) filling materials do contain chemicals that are worth mentioning; however there are few alternatives and certainly these are not as significant as mercury. Many contain fluoride, aluminum and/or Bisphenol-A (BPA). You can ask the dentist for the Material Safety Data Sheet (MSDS) for any products your dentist would like to use. This allows you to know what may be in these products and choose what you feel is appropriate. BPA is said to disrupt the endocrine system, but how much we get from composites isn't clear. Some parents avoid this by choosing a BPA free composite material when they are available.

It is usually acceptable to chelate with stainless steel caps or braces. If you are considering braces, or are concerned about nickel content, you can ask for nickel-free stainless steel products from your child's dentist. You may wish to give the chelator in capsules if possible to reduce contact with these dental metals. If your child has braces that are not nickel free, the content is nominal and is not known to be contraindicated in chelation unless your child has a nickel allergy. In this case you may wish to postpone chelation until their braces have been removed or make sure they have nickel-free dental components.

It is a good idea to avoid fluoride due to its neurotoxic effects. It is very hard to remove fluoride from the body and exposure is cumulative. There is a lot of speculation about the helpful effects of fluoride versus the harm it may cause if ingested. Strong bones and teeth are better made from minerals and healthy diets rather than poor nutrition and fluoride. Strong healthy teeth can be achieved by a natural diet with plenty of Vitamin A, D, K and calcium. While topical fluoride doesn't pose the same risks as ingested fluoride, the main concern is that our children do not rinse well and some do not spit or rinse at all after brushing their teeth, which makes avoiding fluoride toothpastes very important. Luckily there are many natural, fluoride-free types of toothpaste to choose from that contain natural decay deterrents like xylitol. You can research fluoride and make the choice you feel is best for your child.

Parents of ASD children may also have concerns associated with the use of anesthesia by many dentists. Nitrous oxide (gas) is reported as the most problematic because it creates oxidative stress which is already elevated in mercury toxic children. Nitrous oxide depletes enzymes and its use has led to reports of regression symptoms in some ASD children following sedation. Children's liver function also plays a role in their reaction to sedative medications because they do not have the same detoxification capacity that adults do.

Some other inhaled sedatives contain fluoride and are often given with nitrous oxide. (Sevoflurane)

It can be very helpful to find a dentist who is trained to work with children so that sedation drugs are not necessary for your child to have dental work done. If a child must have sedation for a procedure there are other medications that are not associated with the regressions of nitrous oxide.

If this situation applies to your child be sure to discuss all medication options with your dentist or anesthetist. It helps if they are aware of your child's condition as they may be able to offer safer alternatives.

Chapter 11
The Yeast Beast

Fungal infections or yeast are a very common problem for our children. Many parents fear yeast because of the discomfort and behavioral symptoms it can cause. We have witnessed professionals putting off chelation for years focusing solely on treating yeast. Many times parents are told their child has a complicated diagnosis like "intestinal dysbiosis" or some other devastating gut disease that has to be controlled or cured before chelation can begin. This wastes a lot of time and money because it is unnecessary.

The reality is that metals interfere with the immune system's ability to keep opportunistic infections like Candida under control. Although chelation may temporarily increase yeast, it can always be managed. Eventually the immune system will be able to balance and maintain intestinal flora as the toxic metals are reduced. We often say "either treat yeast for a year or two during chelation, or treat yeast for the rest of your child's life." You don't need to postpone or avoid chelation because of yeast.

The digestive system is home to more than 500 different bacterial species. They assist in maintaining healthy intestinal linings, breaking down food, and regulating healthy immune response. According to the currently adopted definition by the World Health Organization, probiotics are: "Live microorganisms, which, when administered in adequate amounts, confer a health benefit on the host".

Probiotics are the first line of defense in an anti-fungal protocol because they help replace these beneficial bacteria. The general recommendation is to take 20-30 billion CFUs or more per day of acidophilus based probiotics. Probiotics are better absorbed on an empty stomach, so try to give them at bedtime or between meals whenever possible.

Testing for yeast is very popular, but not very practical. Many of the tests are notorious for false negatives making parents confused about the symptoms they are seeing and leaving children miserable. Your child's yeast status can change quickly from day to day. Essentially what this means is that even with accurate testing, by the time you receive your child's results their yeast status may have already changed again. So it's our opinion that testing isn't cost effective at this time. It is far easier to base treatment on careful observations of symptoms. By gauging your child's response to anti-fungals and adjusting as needed, you will be able to stay one step ahead.

If your child has any of the symptoms listed in this chapter the most effective approach is to choose an anti-fungal from the list below and begin to use it as suggested. If your child's symptoms improve, or they experience an increase of symptoms followed by relief that is a fairly positive sign that yeast is present. It will be very helpful to learn to recognize your child's individual yeast symptoms so you can manage yeast easily during chelation.

The following are some common symptoms associated with yeast overgrowth that we have seen in children. This list isn't necessarily complete and no one will experience all of these symptoms. It is only intended as a guide. It is possible to experience only one of the listed symptoms and still benefit from yeast treatment. Some parents don't even realize their child had yeast until they saw improvements after treating it, so the proof is often in the pudding.

- White patches in the mouth or coating on the tongue

- Breath that smells like bread or alcohol

- Irritability/defiance, meltdowns, tantrums, anger outbursts

- Only eating or craving starches-intense craving for sweets

- Gas and bloating after meals, or being gassy

- Dark under eye circles

- Tiny red dot rash under arms/groin, sometimes itchy

- Red ring around anus, sometimes itchy

- Constipation

- Itchy inner ears- some ear infections can be yeast

- Sinus congestion, excess mucus, fluid in the ears, thick saliva in the morning, throat mucus

- Frequent stomach pains or digestive problems

- Skin problems like acne, psoriasis, and eczema

- Brain fog-feeling fuzzy headed

- Hyperactivity–"bouncing off the walls"

- Increased obsessive/compulsive behaviors

- Headaches

- Floating/bloated stools, foul smelling stools, gas

- Acting drunk, silly or giddy at inappropriate times

- Increased self stimulation-itchy genitals or anus

Some anti-fungals do destroy naturally occurring probiotics as well as bad bacteria and yeast so it is important to take probiotics to replenish the gut's good bacteria and maintain a healthy balance. Probiotics must be taken 2-4 hours apart from anti-fungals otherwise the anti-fungal will kill the probiotics.

When you first start an anti-fungal protocol ALWAYS start slowly. Once you have seen your child's reaction to the anti-fungal you can increase steadily with moderate doses as needed. The goal is to find the dose that controls yeast. Imagine yeast as little leaky water balloons filled with toxins. When the anti-fungal kills the yeast, the balloon pops and all the toxins are released at once. We refer to this as "die off."

Some die-off is to be expected and generally includes: gas, bloating, or diarrhea. Yeast die-off may include an increase of any symptoms that the yeast produced, like irritability. Extreme die-off may include flu like symptoms and while not life threatening should be avoided because it is very uncomfortable for your child. If this happens lower the dose or stop the anti-fungal until symptoms clear, then start up again at a lower dose.

You can expect that your child may still have some minor signs of yeast when taking anti-fungals but they should be significantly reduced. Curing yeast entirely isn't possible without significant chelation so the goal is to control the symptoms to make your life and your child's a lot more comfortable. When your child's symptoms of yeast are gone, you should stop or significantly reduce the anti-fungals. Most children need a daily maintenance dose for the first year or two of chelation.

You should avoid using any rotational anti-fungal protocols (also called anti-fungal parades), because they can cause resistance to anti-fungals. If resistance happens there are few choices left to fight yeast and you don't want to be in this situation. Most rotational protocols are harsh on the child's gut. We generally see these protocols used with prescription anti-fungals but we have found them unnecessary and they can create a lot of side effects as well as yeast resistance.

The key to anti-fungals is to choose one and use it continually until it is no longer effective at any reasonable dose. Then choose another anti-fungal to use instead. There are also complimenting supplements, that are not anti-fungals but do help in destroying yeast, that can be added to the anti-fungal protocol like biotin and anti-fungal enzymes. These are not always helpful by themselves but can boost an anti-fungal's effectiveness.

Prescription anti-fungals are used by most physicians. They often begin with doses that are too high, which creates terrible die-off symptoms and discourages parents from treating yeast. The other concern is that most toxic children already have compromised or stressed liver function and these medications put even more stress on the liver. We have also noticed that for some reason yeast tends to become resistant to prescription anti-fungals faster-than natural anti-fungals. Since there are natural alternatives readily available that are both effective and have fewer side effects, we do not recommend prescriptions for long term use or in most instances.

The following are dosing suggestions for treating chronic yeast:

Start with ¼-½ of the suggested dose on the bottle of anti-fungal. The first dose can be taken with breakfast and then probiotics at bedtime. If there are no symptoms of die-off or reduction in yeast symptoms you can add a second dose on day two at lunch time. If you see significant die-off symptoms hold the current dose until symptoms subside before you increase the doses again.

Sample Schedule:

- Day one: ½ recommended dose with breakfast. If no symptoms then:

- Day two: ½ recommended dose with breakfast plus a second dose after lunch. If no symptoms:

- Day three: full dose after breakfast and ½ dose after lunch. If you have mild-moderate die-off symptoms then hold the dose for 2-3 days before considering an increase.

Chronic yeast or "yeast flares" are best treated by multi-dosing the anti-fungal 2-3 times a day. If your child experiences a lot of symptoms with a dose increase remember you can reduce the dose slightly until it passes.

Less significant chronic yeast infections can be effectively controlled with one dose of anti-fungal and one dose of probiotics a day. If your child is still having yeast problems on one dose of anti-fungal per day, try adding a second probiotic dose first to see if this helps before you add a second anti-fungal dose.

Some common natural anti-fungals:

- **Grapefruit Seed Extract (GSE)**[11] is most often recommended as a starting anti-fungal because it's very effective and easy to dose. While the liquid form is a little bitter it can be mixed into a citrus juice like orange juice. The tablets have very little taste and can be ground into powder and mixed into any food or drink. GSE is also sold in capsules but these seem to be weaker than tablets or liquids so you may need to use more of it. A small number of children may react negatively to GSE due to phenols, citrus allergies, or some other reason, but most negative reactions are actually from die off caused by starting with too high of a dose.

- **Oil of Oregano (OoO)** is very effective but it has a very strong taste and can be difficult to give to a child who doesn't swallow capsules. The gel capsules are very tiny and can be hidden in applesauce or other soft food to encourage swallowing. OoO is also phenolic so it may not be appropriate for children with phenol issue.

- **Pau D'Arco** is another good anti-fungal. It doesn't appear to be quite as strong as OoO or GSE but it is still very effective especially for children with phenol sensitivity.

- **Candex and Candidase** are enzymes which dissolve the outer cell wall of yeast making it easier for the immune system or anti-fungal to destroy the yeast. They are particularly effective when paired with an anti-fungal and can decrease the amount of anti-fungal required. The enzymes are generally taken on an empty stomach.

---

[11] It should be not be used by someone taking a medication that advised them not to consume grapefruit.

- **Biotin** can be given at 5-10 mg with each meal (3 times per day). While biotin is NOT an antifungal, it can be effective at hindering the mutation of yeast keeping them in their single celled form and therefore easier to kill. It is rarely effective by itself.

Other possible yeast fighters include: Caprylic Acid, Berberines, Garlic, Tannins, etc...

While yeast often strikes fear in most parent's hearts the good news is that with proper treatment yeast is manageable and chelation can be successful. This leads to a real cure for yeast once chelation has removed enough metals for the immune system to function properly again

Chapter 12

Oh So Tired Adrenals

Adrenal fatigue is commonly overlooked in mercury poisoning and certainly in autism, but it can cause significant symptoms like fatigue, anxiety, allergies and frequent illness. The adrenal glands are responsible for many functions in the body including immune function, hormones and thyroid function. Poorly functioning adrenals interfere with the body's normal response to daily stress and illness. If adrenal fatigue is present, it should be treated prior to chelation. Sometimes adrenal fatigue doesn't appear until some months after chelation has begun. This means that your child's adrenals were already struggling and simply need some support in order to handle further stresses, like chelation.

It is important to know that not every child will need adrenal support, but since mercury can impair adrenal function it is very common in our children. There are numerous symptoms of adrenal fatigue and many of them are listed below. Some children may only have one or two symptoms, but still respond well to adrenal support.

Symptoms

- Irritability, meltdowns, whining

- Anxiety, fear, attachment

- Early morning waking especially between 2 am - 4 am (tendency to be wide awake even with little sleep, "tired and wired")

- Allergies

- Asthma

- Inability to fall asleep at night (night owls)

- Morning fatigue

- Frequent illness or inability to recover in a reasonable time from illness

- Sensitivity to light/sound/touch

- Hypersensitive to pain

- Hypoglycemia

- Dizziness upon standing quickly

- Morning nausea or no appetite

- Craving salt

- Low endurance compared to peers

- Constant thirst

- Explosive outbursts or overreaction to situations.

There are a few methods to determine adrenal function that you can do quite easily at home. Since the adrenal glands are responsible for regulating body temperature you can record average daily temperatures to see if they indicate healthy adrenal function. Here is a summary of how to chart temperatures:

- Temperatures should be taken orally or underarm using a glass mercury-free thermometer for 7-10 minutes. Avoid using digital thermometers as they are inaccurate.

- Do this for 5-7 consecutive days and write them down.

- For average daily temperatures take the temperatures three times a day. For example: 9 AM, 12 PM, 3 PM, keep the times consistent from day to day. Avoid taking it until three hours after waking and 30 minutes after a meal or exercise.

- Find the average daily temperatures by adding the three of them together and dividing by three.

Normal average body temperatures should not fluctuate by more than 0.2 degrees up or down from day to day. If you see a fluctuating pattern this indicates poor adrenal function and your child may benefit from adrenal support.

A Doctors Data Inc., Hair Elements test can also be used to determine adrenal fatigue by looking at the minerals section. Dr. Andrew Hall Cutler has details about utilizing the hair test to screen for endocrine issues in his book *Hair Test Interpretations*. While the hair test can indicate a need for adrenal support it cannot be used exclusively to rule out adrenal fatigue. Some children do not show adrenal stress on the hair test but still benefit from adrenal support. Symptoms and temperatures really are the most accurate methods of determining adrenal status.

Sometimes parents ask about the saliva cortisol test. It is not useful for children because currently there are no established pediatric reference ranges. While this test is helpful for adults, until we have accurate ranges for healthy children, it's better to rely on temperature charting and symptoms to figure out what your child needs.

Treating this condition is fairly easy and will provide better health and comfort for your child during the chelation process. Adrenal cortex extract glandular (ACE) is suggested for supporting adrenals in children. ACE nourishes the portion of the adrenal gland that makes cortisol (cortex). This helps the adrenals to make adequate hormones and to heal. It does not contain or provide any significant amount of hormone which is what makes it appropriate for use in children. A whole adrenal glandular is also sold, but is not recommended because it can produce symptoms of high adrenaline, irritability, or hyperactivity in some children. This is because it assists the portion of the adrenal gland that makes adrenaline (medulla) and can result in overproduction.

The general starting dosing suggestions we recommend are as follows:

- Approximately 50-100 mg in the morning for children under 50 pounds.

- Approximately 125-200 mg for children over 50 pounds.

- Approximately 250-350 mg for children over 100 pounds.

If adrenal symptoms return you can either give a second dose or increase the first dose. If the adrenal symptoms are alleviated in the morning, but reappear in the afternoon, consider adding a lunchtime dose. For children in school, it can be given as soon as they get home. ACE can cause difficulty falling asleep in some children if the doses are given after 4 PM, but other children can be dosed as late as 6:00 PM. If your child has difficulties falling asleep consider whether the last dose is being given too late.

Dose increases and suggestions:

- A second dose should be the same amount as the first. For example: a child getting 50 mg in the morning would then add a 50 mg at lunch. Increases are given in small increments.

- Add more if you see adrenal symptoms return.

- It is helpful to multi-dose the glandular through the day to keep adrenal symptoms from reappearing later in the day. Generally a morning, lunchtime and early afternoon dose work best.

- When increasing begin with the morning dose first.

- The proper dose necessary to provide relief from adrenal symptoms varies greatly from child to child. Some children do well with 50-100 mg per day while others need 3-6 capsules per day (250-350 mg each). While less common, we have seen cases when children have needed as much as 7-9 capsules per day.

- Adjust the dose as needed based upon symptoms and condition.

- Adrenal symptoms can increase during a viral infection or chelation. A child may temporarily need more adrenal cortex than they normally take during these times. It may also be helpful to give extra adrenal cortex for a day or two post-round.

- Phosphatidylserine (PS) regulates cortisol rhythm and helps reduce elevations in cortisol production. Children who do not seem to tolerate adrenal cortex may benefit from PS. If a child has symptoms of adrenal fatigue but displays hyperactivity even at low doses of ACE, it is worth considering using PS instead.

Other supplements that can help with adrenal fatigue are: vitamin B5, B6, Vitamin C, and Rhodiola. In many cases these vitamins and herbs are generally not sufficient on their own but can be a helpful part of supporting the adrenals. Children's reactions to these will vary and they may not be appropriate for every child. If they produce negative reactions they should be discontinued.

Chapter 13
Thyroid Conditions

Low thyroid function is quite common in heavy metal toxicity and often goes undetected and untreated by most practitioners. It is important to treat this condition because healthy thyroid function is required for normal growth, brain development, digestion and immunity.

Children do not necessarily gain weight or become overweight as is commonly seen in adults with hypothyroidism. Children tend to be thin, frail or fail to grow properly. A low thyroid can also affect school performance because of fatigue and lack of focus which is sometimes passed off as ADHD (attention deficit hyperactivity disorder).

If your family has a history of autoimmune thyroid conditions such as Hashimoto's or Graves disease, your child has a higher risk of having thyroid problems. In this case your child should be checked for thyroid antibodies along with the full thyroid panel.

Normal thyroid function is dependent on healthy adrenal function. The adrenal glands provide cortisol which helps the thyroid hormones get into the cells so when the thyroid slows down, this pushes the adrenals to work even harder to compensate. If the adrenals are not treated before or in conjunction with the thyroid they will become weaker. This is why any existing adrenal issue needs to be treated before addressing the thyroid. This can be done by starting your child on adrenal cortex (ACE) while waiting to see the practitioner to get thyroid labs.

Symptoms of low thyroid function:

Children with low thyroid function may have some of the following symptoms. Children don't usually display as many symptoms as adults which is often why this condition is not detected until early adulthood.

- May not grow much or have slow growth, "failure to thrive"

- May be tired a lot or, still requiring naps beyond the expected age

- Dry skin, dry hair, hair loss, poor quality nails

- Cold hands and feet

- Constipation and/or colitis

- Thin brittle hair that does not grow well

- Short attention span, difficulty concentrating

- Forgetfulness, poor memory

- Low body temperatures

- Bone or joint pain, feeling weak

- Irritability

- Low mood

- Poor handwriting

- Dental cavities, poor enamel, delayed tooth eruption or loss

Methods of testing:

Serum blood testing that includes Free T4, Free T3, TSH and thyroid antibodies are most useful for determining a thyroid problem when used in conjunction with body temperatures and symptoms. Sometimes labs look fairly well but body temperatures are low indicating there is still a problem.

Most mercury toxic children will not test "out of range" on these thyroid labs. They have what is referred to as sub-clinical thyroid disorder. This means that while they are inside the lab's normal reference ranges, they display symptoms which will only go away with treatment. It is important to understand this lab work properly so that you do not leave your child without the necessary support for proper brain and body development.

Your child should have Free T3 in the upper third of the reference range for optimal health and growth. A TSH level over 1.5 in children indicates that body temperatures, symptoms, and Free T3 levels should be checked to rule out hypothyroidism. The higher the TSH reads above 1.5, the more impaired your child's thyroid is likely to be, because TSH rises when adequate hormone levels are not present.

The following Free T3 reference ranges can be used to help determine if the lab results are adequate for a healthy child.

Suggested Pediatric Reference Ranges for Free T3, Triiodothyronine (FT3), Free (pg/ml) [12]

Age	Male	Female
1-3 days	1.4-4.8	1.4-5.4
4-30days	1.4-5.5	1.5-5.0
1-11mo	2.0-6.9	2.5-6.5
1-5yrs	2.4-6.7	3.0-6.0
6-10yrs	2.9-6.0	2.7-6.2
11-15yrs	3.1-5.9	2.6-5.0
11-18yrs	3.5-5.7	2.8-5.2

Body temperature is also an indication of thyroid function. Low body temperatures indicate that your child's thyroid is under performing and treatment may be needed. The best time to take your child's basal body temperature is first thing in the morning. If possible, it can even be taken just before waking them up for the day. This is most accurately done using a

---

[12] Soldin, Steven J., Antonio Morales, Fedee Albalos, Sara Lenherr, and Nader Rifai. "Pediatric Reference Ranges on the Abbott IMx for FSH, LH, Prolactin, TSH, T4, T3, FreeT4, FreeT3, T-uptake, IgE, and Ferritin." *Clinical Biochemistry* 28.6 (1995): 603-06. Print.

glass (mercury-free) thermometer either orally or axillary (under the arm) for 10 minutes. Optimal basal body temperatures range between 97.8-98° F[13]. A temperature of 97.7° F or less indicates a probable hypothyroid condition. If it is difficult to obtain morning basal temperatures you can chart your child's average daily temperatures instead. You want to see optimal average daily temperatures of 98.6°F[14].

Hair Testing can sometimes reveal glimpses into thyroid function. Dr. Cutler's book on *Hair Test Interpretations* provides detailed information on what to look for if you would like to learn about it. While a hair test can show thyroid problems before lab tests do, it cannot rule out a thyroid problem. In most cases our most reliable means are temperature charting and serum thyroid panels.

Treatment:

It is important to treat low thyroid function because it will lead to many health issues including growth problems and loss of IQ in children which may not be reversible. Hypothyroidism is usually treated with thyroid hormone replacement and then follow-up blood work is done to monitor hormone levels to keep them in a safe healthy range.

Desiccated thyroid medication is recommended because it is the most bio-identical option for replacing our natural supply of thyroid hormone. Most mainstream physicians prefer to use synthetic T4 medication (Levothyroxine). This will normalize TSH levels but often does not relieve all the thyroid symptoms.

The two most common brands of desiccated thyroid are called Armour Thyroid and Nature-Throid, but there are others that are fine also. These

---

[13] 36.5° Celsius

[14] 37.0° Celsius

medications will normalize TSH levels but they also work better to alleviate most hypothyroid symptoms. Treatment with desiccated thyroid should always be monitored under the supervision of a doctor. Usually a moderate dose of desiccated thyroid is started for six weeks and repeat serum labs are done to determine if the dose needs to be raised.

If your child needs thyroid medication it's helpful to know the symptoms of excess thyroid hormone so you can report these to your child's doctor and reduce the dose if necessary.

Symptoms of an overactive or over-medicated thyroid include:

- High body temps of 99° F or more

- Rapid or fast resting pulse

- Shaking arms, hands, feeling jittery

- Loss of appetite

- Inability to sleep, hyperactivity

These symptoms are not common when reasonable doses of desiccated thyroid are used and follow up blood work is done to monitor appropriate dosing.

Most children will need regular monitoring of their thyroid levels until the metals have been reduced enough for their thyroid to function normally again. When mercury is the cause of the thyroid malfunction, chelation will allow you to wean your child from medication so that they do not need to be on it for life.

It is important to know that lab work does not always match patient symptoms because mercury can block thyroid hormone receptors. When that happens your child may have normal levels of circulating hormone, but it isn't getting into the cells. This is why it's important to consider symptoms and body temperatures when determining thyroid status and not rely solely on lab work.

Optimal thyroid function results when symptoms are gone and TSH is 1.5 or less with T3 in the upper third of the range. Some children need a dose adjustment periodically. This is more common in the spring and fall when thyroid function naturally changes. It is important to work with a doctor and use subsequent lab work to monitor the treatment.

Special Considerations: Another important factor to consider in hypothyroidism is the thyroid antibodies. Thyroid peroxidase antibody (TPO) and Thyroglobulin antibody (TgAb) are indicators that the immune system is attacking the thyroid. The higher these levels, the more significant the current attack is. In cases of autoimmune hypothyroidism it is important to remember that serum thyroid hormone levels may not be as accurate in reflecting the true levels of thyroid hormone accessible to your child's body.

If you have a child with autoimmune hypothyroidism you can expect an up and down fluctuation in their thyroid symptoms in relation to what the immune system is doing. Some things that help this condition in addition to taking thyroid medication are; following a gluten-free diet, treating gut bacteria and parasites and addressing chronic viral conditions in the body. If you have autoimmune hypothyroidism these antibodies may have been present during pregnancy where they cross the placenta causing your child to develop autoimmune thyroid disease.

Autoimmune thyroid conditions can sometimes be improved by maintaining a gluten-free diet. Thyroid and gluten proteins look similar to the immune system and for some children with leaky gut; their body will attack the thyroid on its hunt to eliminate gluten in the blood stream. You may wish to avoid feeding your child foods or supplements with soy if they are hypothyroid because soy acts to block thyroid hormones.

Iodine is often recommended to treat thyroid dysfunction, however high doses are not usually good for autoimmune hypothyroidism. In some individuals too much iodine has been reported to cause autoimmune attacks. If your child is not autoimmune a reasonable dose of 250 mcg per day of iodine in the diet can be helpful if they are deficient. In more significant cases iodine alone is insufficient and generally does not replace the need for thyroid hormones. Do not spend too long trying iodine if your child has hypothyroid labs.

Other supplements you should consider, that are important in thyroid function are adequate Vitamin D and selenium for thyroid hormone conversion. Most people who are hypothyroid are deficient in Vitamin D so this should be tested by your child's doctor. Misuse of calcium in the body is also common in hypothyroidism so additional calcium and vitamin K may be needed in order to maintain bone, gut, teeth and liver health.

Chapter 14
Tummy Troubles

It is very common for our children to have gut and digestive issues. There is a misconception circulating in the autism community that your child's gut must be healed before chelation. In our experience, the gut can never heal while the body is toxic. Chelation improves gut function and it is preferable to work on improving the gut while chelating. We have previously discussed how to treat and control yeast but this is only one component to healing the gut. Improving gut function may also include things like making changes to the diet, as well as treating bacteria and parasites.

Constipation is a frequent problem that many of our children experience. The most common cause of constipation with ASD children is the overgrowth of Candida (yeast) in the gut. If yeast is under control and constipation is still a problem you will want to investigate other possible causes like: diet, digestion, dehydration, thyroid function, or bile flow.

Many children with ASD have difficulty digesting casein or dairy proteins which are found in things like milk or cheese. When these foods are eliminated and replaced with dairy-free substitutes (like nut milks) their constipation resolves. Some children can tolerate raw/fermented cow or goat milk. Other children have a true intolerance to casein and must stick to a strict casein-free diet. It is also important that adequate fruit and vegetables are a part of your child's diet to provide enough natural fiber for digestion. Many ASD children self-limit their food choices and may not eat a large enough variety of these foods. You can improve this by using smoothies with fresh or powdered greens and fruits.

Adequate water intake is important for normal bowel function. Some ASD children do not recognize the need to drink or eat regularly and may need to be reminded to drink enough liquids each day.

If yeast seems to be controlled and dietary modifications haven't helped you may want to rule out hypothyroidism which is known to cause chronic constipation that doesn't improve with dietary changes.

Low liver bile flow is another factor in sluggish bowel function that can cause constipation. Milk thistle helps the liver and gall bladder produce more bile which improves digestion. Because mercury can inactivate some enzymes, you might also consider giving your child additional digestive enzymes which help to break down food in the stomach so it is digested more completely.

The following suggestions can help prevent and alleviate constipation:

- Make sure your child is drinking enough fluids.

- Give extra magnesium which usually produces a stool within a few hours by drawing water to the colon. (for this purpose magnesium sulfate is a good choice)

- Rule out food intolerance to dairy/gluten. You can do this with an elimination trial diet.

- Don't give too much extra fiber because this can make large and bulky, hard to pass stools. Your child should not strain or have pain; this may create a stretched colon if it happens a lot.

- Natural senna tea/products can be purchased and used in small doses. This should produce a stool within 12 hours.

- Prune juice or eating prunes can promote regularity.

- Probiotics: these often resolve chronic issues in many children.

- Increasing (non-buffered) Vitamin C can help produce loose stools.

- Digestive enzymes to insure food is properly broken down and moving through the digestive tract.

- Avoid refined foods, they don't contain good fiber and our bodies are not designed to digest hydrogenated oils or other chemicals.

- OxyPowder: This product works well for promoting regular bowel function. (Miralax is not recommended for our children).

- For severe constipation lasting days, you can give a glycerin suppository for children or contact your child's doctor. It is best to use the above listed options to prevent severe constipation.

Diarrhea or loose stools are the other common gut issue in ASD children. There are many interventions that can help address this problem. Chronic loose stools sometimes indicate a food allergy or sensitivity. Allergies or intolerance to gluten, casein, soy or other allergens should be investigated and the offending food removed from the diet if necessary.

If you have already removed known allergens from your child's diet but they still continue to have loose stools the following factors should be considered:

- The dose of probiotics may be too high.

- The dose of anti-fungals or anti-bacterial may be too high.

- The dose of magnesium, vitamin C, or taurine may be too high. Each of these supplements is known to cause loose stools. This is one of the reasons they can be used to treat constipation. If you recently increased one of them, suspect this as a cause if there are no other signs of illness like foul smell, odd color.

- Viral infection which usually comes with foul smell and/or odd color. Giving activated charcoal and anti-virals during the flu can be helpful. Avoid giving activated charcoal at the same time with supplements and never during a round of chelation.

- Bacterial infections which also present with odd stool color and odor. They can be treated with things like Goldenseal, Uva Ursi and/or Culturelle.

The symptoms often associated with bacterial gut infections are; defiant behavior, anger, meltdowns, diarrhea, aggression, violence (biting, kicking, hitting, etc.) and foul, smelly stool. Some children may also have a bloated abdomen. The treatment we have found most effective for bacteria is to use Goldenseal at 250-500 mg, three times per day for up to two weeks, no longer. In addition, Culturelle probiotics are helpful at a minimum of 3 capsules dosed at least 4 hours away from any anti-fungals or anti-bacterials. You can alternate Goldenseal with other bacterial fighters such as Uva Ursi or cranberry, etc.

Goldenseal is just as, if not more, effective than prescription antibiotics like Flagyl or Vancomycin. We do not recommend these prescriptions because they are very hard on the liver which is often compromised in mercury poisoning.

Parasites also affect bowel function causing symptoms like diarrhea, constipation or irritable bowel. Parasitic infections are acquired naturally through foods, other humans or animals. Anyone can get them by playing in soil or walking outside barefoot. Pets can carry parasites and transmit them to your child if your pets are not treated for parasites periodically. Parasites cause disease or illness in our bodies. They contribute to nutritional deficiencies, malabsorption and intestinal dysfunction. Parasites also release waste products into your child's body that can affect their health.

Symptoms of parasitic infections vary and may not be clear in every case. If your child has never had a parasite cleanse its more likely they may have parasites.

These symptoms are common but if they do not resolve with other therapies parasites cleansing may help[15]:

- Diarrhea

- Chronic constipation

- Gas and bloating

---

[15] The safety of parasite cleanses during pregnancy has not been established. Consult your doctor in this situation.

- Explosive diarrhea or bowel movements very shortly after eating

- Abdominal pains

- Mucus in stool

- Leaky gut

- Nausea

- Hemorrhoids

- Burning in the stomach

- Bloody stool

- Fatigue

- Allergies

- Itchy nose

- Itchy anus

- Skin conditions

- Eczema

- Itchy or crawling skin

- Mood swings

- Nervousness

- Depression

- Anxiety

- Teeth grinding that does not improve with mineral supplements

- Bed wetting

- Night mares or bad dreams, waking during the night

- Uncontrollable hunger despite eating normal meals

- Body aches or joint pains

- Hypoglycemia

- Anemia

Treatment for parasites is relatively easy and cost effective. Treatment is safe, affordable and the simplest way to address the problem.

If your child has parasites, they will display a few symptoms or improvements in the first week of parasite herbs. There are three main herbs used in parasite cleanses that are known to address all three stages of a parasite life cycle. These are wormwood, walnut hull[16], and cloves. This combination of herbs kills the parasite adult, larvae and eggs. There are other herbs used in various products that are effective also. You should choose a product formulated for children.

Herbs should be started at a low dose and slowly increased over 3-4 days reaching the recommended dose on the bottle. Remember to adjust the dose for a child if using an adult product. Starting slowly will reduce the die-off reaction. It is best to use the herbs for 38 days, beginning four days before the full moon and ending four days after the next full moon. This will cover the full life cycle of the parasite and insure all the eggs have been killed. A cleanse can be done a few times a year or anytime there is a return of symptoms. There should be a break of 30 or more days between cleanses.

---

[16] Those allergic to tree nuts should consider if using walnut hull would be problematic for them.

Symptoms that occur during cleansing usually appear during the first 7-10 days.

These are the most common ones reported:

- More frequent stools (2-3 times a day) in the first week

- Symptoms of irritability

- Temporary depression, moodiness or brain fog

- Fatigue

- Headache

In some cases your child may not have any side effects but, a strong reaction usually means they have a significant parasitic infection, in which case a parasite cleanse is needed. Antioxidants and liver support can be helpful if your child's die-off reactions are bothersome.

The herbal tinctures for parasite cleanses have a strong taste so you should try to mix them into some kind of liquid or food if they cannot be swallowed in capsules. Children with strong oral sensory issues can use a trans-dermal application of the parasite tincture. You can do this by applying the liquid to the bottom of their feet at bedtime.

Additional points about parasites:

- Parasites have a life cycle and their egg laying is active around the full moon. Children who get hyper or have erratic behavior around the full moon usually have parasites.

- Cleansing is not invasive and does not usually produce diarrhea. Some children will experience various symptoms during the first week but should be able to conduct normal daily activities. In many cases parasite herbs reduce or eliminate yeast. If die-off symptoms are extreme you can use activated charcoal making sure not to use it near herbs, supplements and never during a round of chelation.

- It is helpful to drink plenty of water, although bowel function usually improves when taking herbs. In most cases there is no need to use enemas or laxatives however if your child becomes constipated they can help relieve it.

Chapter 15
Juggling Supplements

We can divide supplements into three basic categories according to importance during the recovery process.

Support Supplements are things you give your child to support chelation which all mercury toxic children need to be on provided they tolerate them. These are the four basic or essential supplements we discussed earlier: Magnesium, Vitamin C, Zinc, and Vitamin E.

General Health Supplements begin with a good multivitamin/mineral which has the right balance of B vitamins (some children don't tolerate B's), also includes Cod Liver Oil and probiotics. (Milk thistle may also be considered in this category).

Need Based Supplements are given on an "as needed basis" only. This category includes things like adrenal cortex extract (ACE), anti-fungals, enzymes, thyroid support, high dose B's, antibacterials, neuro-support, etc... These are supplements added which you only keep if there is a positive indication that they are helping.

When first introducing begin with the Support Supplements then add the General Health Supplements. Wait a minimum of three days between each new supplement (a multi-vitamin is considered one new supplement unless your child reacts to it, then you get to try introducing each ingredient individually). When you get to the Need Based Supplements, you only introduce the things your child demonstrates a possible need for based on signs and symptoms and you may need to take more than three days between each new introduction. You might find it helpful to keep a written record of what supplements, doses and responses you see so that you can keep track of what is helpful and what is not.

When removing supplements this process gets reversed. Never remove all your child's supplements at once as this often results in negative reactions or regressions. Begin with the Need Based Supplements and remove them one at a time watching for regressions and understanding the general reason the supplement would be needed so that you know what to watch for. This is particularly helpful if your child is on a very long list of supplements and you aren't sure what is working anymore. As your child progresses with chelation and their metal burden is reduced they will require less and less additional support.

Chapter 16
Additional Supplements

This is a list of some of the common supplements that you might use with your child in biomedical therapy to address various symptoms and conditions or simply to provide optimized nutrition. These are not supplements required for chelation. The doses are only guidelines based upon what we have seen working for our children and what seems reasonable. Just like with most things, too much or too little can cause problems. We suggest using reasonable doses as outlined and doing some of your own research to determine if your child needs any of these.

This list is alphabetized and not in order of importance. Your child **will not** need all of these.

Name	Dose	Purpose/ Additional Information
5HTP	50-200 mg per day	Anti-depressant helps anxiety, insomnia.
Adrenal Cortex Extract	Refer to chapter 12 for detail dosing guidelines	Anxiety, OCD, Sensitivity to light/sound/touch. Adrenal Cortex Extract glandular is preferred, not whole adrenal tissue.
Activated Charcoal	¼-½ cap to start	Absorbs yeast die-off, good for flu/gut bugs, food infractions. NEVER give within 45 minutes of supplements or on chelation rounds.

Active Folate-5-MTHF	Unknown	Needed by people who cannot reduce folic acid, MTHFR gene mutation.
Aloe Vera Juice	Follow mfg. dosing	Helps heal gut, reduces inflammation.
Astragalus	Follow mfg. dosing	Immune support. Liquid tincture is more potent.
Beta Glucan	Follow mfg. dosing	Immune Booster.
Biotin	Start as 400 mcg per day, 5-10 mg per meal	This B vitamin helps the body fight yeast. It is not an antifungal.
B Complex	2.5-25 mg four times a day	Anti stress, supports adrenals, helps with brain function Not everyone tolerates B's. Look for yeast-free forms.
B1 thiamine B2 riboflavin	See B complex.	
B6 pyridoxine	25-50 mg a day	Adrenal support. Long term high dose B6 can deplete B2 and cause peripheral neuralgia.

B12 cobalamin	40-60 mcg per kg sublingual dosed 3-4 times per day	Helps methylation. Some will benefit from either the methyl form or the hydroxy form. MB12 shots are not recommended as they have been shown to elevate cobalt levels. Can increase yeast.
Boron	1-2 mg per day	Helps with building bone.
Calcium	1-3 yrs 500 mg 4-8 yrs 800 mg 9-18 yrs 1300 mg	Builds bones, needed for tooth enamel, especially in CF kids. Ask for assay of product; pick one with the lowest lead content. Any brand that is tested.
Caprylic Acid	800-1200 mg per day	Anti-fungal.
Carnitine	500-2000 mg per day	Helps with energy by acting on mitochondria and can help children with muscle tone problems.
Carnosine	600-1200 mg per day	Helps some ASD children with seizures, but has had adverse effects on some kids. Can cause irritability and sadness. Discontinue if this happens.
Citicoline	500-2000 mg per day. In evenly divided dosages.	Protect neurons, improves signal transmission and improves focus.

Chromium	100-200 mcg with meals	For hypoglycemia.
Choline	see phosphatidyl choline	Focus, concentration, helps the hippocampus work well but can worsen epileptic conditions. Choline bitrate does not survive the stomach, phosphatidylcholine or lecthin does.
Cod Liver Oil	1-6 Tbsp. per day	Provides A, D and DHA for brain function and focus. Helps promote normal dental development. Must be mercury/metal/PCB free.
Colostrum	Follow mfg. dosing	Immune booster/modulator.
Copper	Only in case of copper deficiency, otherwise avoid it.	Contraindicated unless there is serum verified deficiency.
CoQ-10	30-200 mg per day	Antioxidant that helps counter mercury damage.
DMG	44lb 125-375 mg 66lb 190-560 mg 88lb 250-750 mg 110lb 300-900 mg	Improve language, eye contact, energy. Makes some kids hyper, if so then use TMG. It is a methyl donor.

Echinacea	½ cap 3x a day or per instruction on product.	Immune support, helps fend off illness or colds.
EFA's (essential fatty acids)	1-3 tbsp per day	Focus, brain function, reduce inflammation, and protect nervous system, helps skin problems, dyspraxia. Flax, fish oils, coconut oil.
Elderberry	Follow mfg. directions	Immune Support, good for respiratory infections.
EpiCor	¼-½ cap or more	Immune booster. Does not cause yeast
GABA	50-100 mg 3x a day for 50 pd child	Helpful for language, anxiety, mood swings, insomnia and seizures. Can make you sleepy in higher doses. Any brand, also comes sublingual.
Garlic Oil	500-3000 mg per day	Anti-fungal, Anti-bacterial.
Glutathione	Transdermal only in rare cases for low cysteine children, generally not beneficial	Oral is destroyed in the gut. It's contraindicated for high cysteine children. Never IV or oral.
Goldenseal Root	250-500 mg 2 x a day	Excellent for bacteria, also helps with yeast. Standardized brands are best.

Grapefruit Seed Extract	Start slowly with ¼ to ½ tablet per day	Anti-fungal, anti-bacterial. Requires probiotics and take them 4+ hours after the GSE. May not be suitable for children with significant phenol problems or slow liver phase one.
Glycine	1000-1500 mg	Calming, helps heal the gut, boost glutathione.
Inositol	Work up to 1000 mg a day. For OCD issues, up to 9 grams per day.	Helps the health of cell membranes, can also be used to boost immune system. Antidepressant often used to reduce high calcium or lower iron levels.
Iodine	150-250 mcg per day	Helps thyroid health.
Iron	Generally not recommended	Mercury toxicity often causes low iron in the body in order to reduce oxidative stress. Taking iron usually does not correct the problem when mercury is causing it and often makes your child feel worse. Consider cooking in cast iron pots/pans or using powdered greens and natural food sources of iron if low iron levels are detected on serum.

L-Glutamine	1-4 + grams per day for adults	Improves brain function, helps heal gut, and boosts immune function. Can cause ammonia in certain people.
Lecithin(Phosphatidylcholine)	1500-9000 mg per day	Helps liver, brain and digestion. Generally derived from soy, but soy free versions can be found.
L-Lysine	1-2 grams per day	Anti-viral.
Magnesium	300-800 mg should be divided into four daily doses	Needed for muscle function, constipation, tics, phenol issues, and insomnia. Citrate, malate, glycinate forms are best. Avoid oxide, poorly absorbed.
Manganese	Not recommended in mercury toxicity	Manganese should only be used when determined deficiency is present and in low doses. It increases oxidative stress when present with mercury.
Melatonin	1-2 mg or less given ½ hour before bed	Helps with sleep problems, good for the immune system. Promotes regulation of sleep/wake cycles in adrenal fatigue. Any brand, some find timed release better for those who fall asleep well but wake up in the middle of the night.

Milk Thistle	¼-½ cap or 20-80 mg per dose	Liver support! Helps the liver heal and function better. It should say "Silymarin" in the ingredient list.
Molybdenum	5-20 mcg per pound divided 4 x a day	It is used to lower copper; also helps reduce the symptoms of mercury.
NAC (N-Acetyl Cysteine)	No more than 100-200 mg total, per day, while chelating, in divided doses.	Liver support; tends to feed yeast. Only for low-cysteine children.
N Acetyl Carnitine	See carnitine.	
N-acetyl glucosamine (NAG)	200-500 mg	Supposed to help gut. Usually derived from seafood sources, this might be an allergen concern.
Niacin as **Niacinamide** (B3)	1-2 grams a day in divided doses	Start low; the body will dump what it doesn't need. It is helpful for chemical sensitivity and autoimmunity. Do not use Niacin. Niacin is hard on the liver.
Olive Leaf Extract	500-1500 mg per day	Antiviral, antibacterial. Can flare yeast.

Oregano Oil	As much as needed	Antifungal, Antibacterial. Also very useful for asthma flares, shortness of breath.
Pantothenic Acid (B5)	200+ mg given a few times a day	Excellent for adrenal support.
Phosphatidyl-choline (lecthin)	1500-9000 mg per day	Helps liver, brain and digestion. Generally derived from soy, but soy free versions can be found.
Phosphatidyl-serine	100-200 mg per day	Improve concentration, focus, and mood, modulate cortisol levels.
Pycnogenol/ grape seed extract	25-200mg per day	Antioxidant not to be confused with grape**fruit** extract.
SAMe	5-15 mg/kg per day	Not usually helpful.
Selenium	1-2 mcg per pound divided into four	Antioxidant supports thyroid function. Avoid selenium made from yeast. Use selenomethionine form.
Taurine	500 mg-2000 mg per day	Liver support, focus, calming.

TMG	44lb 150-500 mg 66lb 250-800 mg 88lb 350-1050 mg 110lb 450-1300 mg 132lb 550-1600 mg	Improve language, eye contact, methyl donor. Alternate to DMG, good for increasing energy.
Transfer Factor	Follow dose on the bottle.	Immune modulation.
Vanandium	2-5 mg per day	For hypoglycemia
Vitamin A	10,000-25,000 IU per day for maintenance as much as 500-1000 IU per pound when needed[17]	Helps with visual stims and language, anti-viral, children don't convert beta carotene. Good for immune, gut and neurological support.
Vitamin C	250-500 mg per dose given 4x day	Antioxidant, immune booster. If corn is an issue, make sure it's not made from corn. There are some nice cassava or tapioca forms available. If corn free vitamin C is a problem consider a possible oxalate issue.

---

[17] Watch for vitamin A toxicity when giving higher doses. One of the first signs of too much A is dry chapped lips. High doses of vitamin C and a high protein diet help protect against vitamin A toxicity.

Vitamin E	400-800 IU per day	Antioxidant, D-alpha tocopherol is the natural form, not dl-alpha. Higher doses of E best used with 1-3 mg of Vitamin K.
Vitamin D	400-1000IU per day	Support immune function, prevents flu, needed for bone formation D3 only. D2 is made using radiation.
Vitamin K	1-5 mg day	Needed for bones and clotting, helps get rid of cavities, K1 or K2.
Zinc	Weight in pounds plus 20 mg divided, 2 or more times per day (30 lb child would take 50 mg total)	Helps with PICA (chewing on clothes or putting objects in mouth) Immune support, lowering copper recommended forms: glycinate, picolinate, monomethionine, chelate, and citrate.

Chapter 17
Choosing the Right Diet

Children with ASD benefit from dietary interventions which help improve gut function, behavior and overall health. Some children have true food allergies to things like gluten, casein or soy. Other children have food intolerance due to digestive issues but do not demonstrate a true allergy on lab testing. In either case it is often beneficial to remove these foods from the diet until adequate chelation has been done.

The easiest place to start is by feeding your child an all natural diet that is free of processed foods. Then you can begin to investigate what other foods may be problematic for your child. Testing can be done for children who are suspected of being intolerant or allergic to specific foods. Sometimes eliminating foods indicated as problematic on the test makes a big difference, other times it does not appear to be helpful so you will have to watch for improvements when removing a food to determine if it is necessary to restrict it long term.

Removing chemicals, food additives and sugar will benefit most of our children. Many common food additives are known to have a negative effect on children's behavior and most of these foods are not very nutritious. These chemicals are another burden on an already toxic body.

Diets are helpful but they do not cure heavy metal toxicity. They can greatly improve quality of life while you work to remove the metals through chelation. We suggest choosing the most appropriate diet based on the indications below and then doing a diet trial. If you carefully note your child's reactions, you will be able to determine if a given diet offers enough quality of life improvement to continue it. Some of the most common diets found helpful with ASD children are listed below.

- **Weston A Price (WAP)-** This is a very nourishing diet which focuses on high quality fats, nutrient dense bone broths, and the elimination of processed food and food additives/chemicals.

Indications: Chemical sensitivity, malnourishment or failure to thrive, cholesterol imbalance, poor bone development or dental health. **Diet Trial:** 2 months.

- **Low Sulfur*-**This diet reduces excess monothiols (sulfur molecule) in the blood, by restricting high sulfur foods like broccoli, eggs, and dairy. Sulfur feeds yeast so reducing it will be helpful in controlling yeast issues. **Indications:** Difficulty controlling yeast even with large amounts of anti-fungals and probiotics. This diet seems to work when yeast seems to acclimate to any anti-fungal used within a short period of time (it is common to quickly acclimate to Rx anti-fungals and does not necessarily indicate a sulfur issue). Children with increased hyperactivity, meltdowns, self-restricting to sulfur foods. **Diet trial:** 1-2 weeks

- **Casein-Free (CF)-**This diet is the complete elimination of all dairy foods and requires strict adherence as small infractions are enough to reverse the benefit. **Indications:** Demonstrated intolerance to dairy, sinus congestion, night terrors, constipation diarrhea and mucus in the stool. **Diet Trial:** 1-2 weeks

- **Gluten-Free (GF)-**This diet requires the complete elimination of all gluten grains including; wheat, barley and rye. You have to strictly avoid all gluten. This is the only diet which must be followed when gluten allergy is detected on testing, regardless of its effects on behavior because gluten has a strong autoimmune component. **Indications:** Self-limiting to gluten foods. Positive test for gluten antibodies indicates a 100% gluten-free diet; no need for trial. **Diet Trial:** 4 weeks

- **The Feingold Diet-**This diet eliminates artificial coloring, flavoring, preservatives, phenolic foods and salicylates. It is fairly easy to implement and benefits a great majority of children who have phenol and salicylate problems. **Indications:** Hyperactivity, aggressiveness, red cheeks or ears, sometimes dark under-eye circles, ADHD focus issues. Epsom salts baths may help the liver process chemicals in these children. **Diet Trial:** 1-2 weeks.

- **SCD/BED/GAPS-**This diet eliminates complex and includes only monosaccharides like fruit, meat, a vegetables. It can be helpful for reducing gut inf controlling yeast. **Indications:** Difficulty controllir gut issues. **Diet Trial:** 1-2 weeks

- **Allergy Elimination/Rotation-**This diet removes all food sensitivities and rotating the remaining tolerated foods every four days. This is helpful in cases of extreme, multiple food sensitivities. If no reaction is seen to removing or reintroducing foods there is no need to continue. **Indications:** In cases of overactive immune reaction, leaky gut or when a child becomes reactive to any food ingested on a regular basis. **Diet trial:** 2-4 weeks (reintroduce only one new food item at a time).

The key to diet is to optimize nutrition and reduce symptoms while chelating to get the metals out. You do not need to have a diet in place prior to beginning supplementation or chelation. Support for implementing a diet can be found online or through websites and message forums.

Note: Cysteine is an essential amino acid and is helpful for many body processes. Sulfur foods are rich in the amino acids methionine and cysteine. Sulfur is a monothiol meaning that, when in excess, it can attach to heavy metals and "bounce them around" without actually causing them to exit the body in any significant amount. This creates behavior issues and a lot of yeast issues for some children.

It is theorized that a large percentage of children who benefit from the GFCF diet are actually benefiting from the low cysteine aspect of the diet. An opiate or autoimmune reaction to gluten and casein require strict adherence, however, children differ in the amount of sulfur they can tolerate. Since the tolerance to sulfur varies, it only makes sense to investigate sulfur status first. This can be done by doing the low sulfur diet trial for 1-2 weeks then reintroducing eggs, and beans, if you see no reaction after 2-3 days, introduce dairy. If you see a decline in behavior only after the dairy was reintroduced you know that your child has intolerance to dairy rather than a problem with sulfur.

Chapter 18
Immune Function

Infants are born without fully functioning immune systems. In early life babies are protected from disease by their mother's milk which contains any antibodies Mom has built up over the years. It takes a couple of years for a child to develop a fully functional generalized immune system. Having a solid, working and balanced immune function the child's body is now ready to begin forming specific antibodies to fight off a variety of viral assaults. This is one of the wisdom's behind nursing for the first two years of an infant's life as seen in a variety of traditional cultures.

Vaccines force the body into overdrive making it swing wildly back and forth between two extremes. Sometimes it will get stuck in one mode or another.

It is very common to find viral issues in our children because of this early tampering with the normal development of the immune system and because mercury specifically damages immune response.

Mary's daughter has always been sickly. As a child she suffered from one virus or infection after another and was constantly on prescription antibiotics. She even spent time in the hospital once or twice because she just couldn't get over a particular illness.

Susie's son was a lively boy. He never came down with any illness. Even when the rest of the family was vomiting with the stomach flu or struggling with a bad cold Tommy never got sick. One winter his brother and sister both had chicken pox and a month later they each took their turn with strep throat but Tommy has never had so much as the sniffles.

Believe it or not both of these children suffer from immune dysfunction and may need to do an anti-viral protocol as part of their recovery process. While Mary's daughter obviously is struggling and unable to fight off the everyday viruses effectively, Susie's son Tommy's immune system isn't even trying. He is coming into contact with the same viruses as the rest of the family, but his immune system is asleep at the wheel leaving the viruses to multiply at whim.

It is important not to go after viruses too soon because your child needs a functioning immune system in order to keep the viruses at bay. It takes around a year of chelation (50+ rounds) to get enough metals out so that a viral protocol can be effective at controlling the virus and not make your child miserable in the process. We do not recommend going after viruses if your child is still struggling with yeast.

It is possible that after a significant amount of chelation your child's immune system can kick in and begin to get rid of viruses without ever needing outside support in the form of a full viral protocol.

If yeast is well controlled and you have done a significant amount of chelation but your child still exhibits some of the following symptoms, it may be a good time to consider going after viruses:

- Your child actually functions better when they are ill or have a fever.

- Your child has low muscle tone or motor problems (especially if on only one side of their body).

- Temporary improvement in function or behavior while taking antibiotics

- Some common blood count readings which indicate viral issue: are routinely high B cell count, low NK cell count, and an irregular ratio of T-helper cells to T-suppressor cells.

Winter may not be the best time to go after viruses because it is cold and flu season. We recommend starting this when you feel your child is at their least susceptible time.

- Choose three or more antivirals from the list along with an immune modulator.

- Introduce one at a time beginning with a low dose and increasing until you reach the recommended dose on the bottle for children.

- Once you have them all on board you will continue for 3-4 months provided you see gains.

- You may need to repeat this process a few times until there are no longer any reactions to the anti-virals.

- You may also need to play around with the combination a bit depending upon how many and which viruses are causing issues.

Some of the positive results seen with antiviral protocols are better or more stabilized mood, increase in language skills, and better social skills. Sometimes the benefits are as subtle as an overall increase in motivation or maturity.

It is common for an antiviral protocol to cause some yeast flare even if it was previously controlled. You may need to increase anti-fungals while controlling viruses, if yeast is too difficult to control, or if your child is miserable, discontinue the antivirals. You can try again after another 25-30 more rounds of chelation.

Immune Modulators:

- Colostrum

- Beta Glucan

- Epicor

- Vitamin D3

- Lactoferrin

- Thymic Protein A

Antivirals:

- Lauricidin

- Elderberry

- Astragalus Root (not more than two weeks per month)

- Echinacea (not more than two weeks per month)

- Olive Leaf Extract

- Vitamin C

- Vitamin A

- Virastop

- Cat's Claw

- Turmeric or Curcumin

- Garlic

- Licorice

- Zinc

- St John's Wort

- Inositol

- Inosine

- Oil of Oregano

- Transfer Factor

Note: The advantage of using natural antivirals over prescription ones like Valtrex, is that they target a multitude of viruses rather than just a single strain. This gives your child a superior broad spectrum attack which should reduce the time it takes to complete the process. If your child is on any prescription medicines, especially psychotropics or anti-seizure medications, be sure to check for interactions before using any herbals.

Chapter 19
On the Road to Recovery

Autism is never easy for any family or any child. We have been there with our own children and we remember how it was when we started out. There were so many facets to biomedical therapy and it seemed daunting trying to learn it all. We haven't forgotten how difficult it was then and how important it was to know that there were other parents out there who understood what we were going through.

Autism is definitely a challenge and none of us expects to travel this road, but you can manage with the right tools. There is hope and there is healing in autism. Children do learn to speak, they do regain eye contact and they do come back to their parents. This road isn't easy and it does have its ups and downs. Sometimes you make progress, other times it seems like maybe nothing much is happening. Then one day you wake up and your child is doing something you never thought they could do. That confirms that all this work you've done, all this learning, chelation and managing supplements really is paying off.

We have found that the protocols in this book become a life style rather than a therapy. It seems that mercury, immune dysfunction, and endocrine problems tend to run in families. If your child was susceptible, usually parents and siblings are too. Before you know it everyone is eating better, taking vitamins and removing metals. In a few years time you realize how much healthier your family is and that's what came from autism. Autism demands that we change. With a positive attitude and the right information it can lead to a healthier life for the family, not just your autistic child. When we become more informed, and proactive we discover that we do have the power to do better, to BE better.

We have done our best to gather the most useful therapies, present them in an easy to follow manner, so we can teach you what we have learned. So we can help you help your child. We know what it's like when your kitchen counter resembles a vitamin shop.

We know how hard it is to get up at night, week after week, to give chelators. But we also know that if we could go back and do it all over again, we would. Getting our children back is worth any sacrifices we've made to do these therapies. So with these thoughts, and this book to guide you, we wish you well on your road to recovery.

About the Authors

Jan's Story

My son's story is like that of many which began with symptoms following vaccinations in early infancy. My son seemed to be settling in just fine as a newborn. He was eating and sleeping well until his 2 month vaccines. This was only the beginning of what would be a gradual slow road to autism.

After his vaccines he began to cry all the time. He would scream at night and it seemed like he never slept. By the time he was 6 months old I was exhausted from spending most of my nights rocking him. As an infant he screamed when riding in the car. As he grew it was clear that many of his behaviors were peculiar. He was obsessed with the heat registers in the wall, switches and he used to escape from the house. Much of his speech was advanced but also included non-sense or chatter that sounded like a foreign language. He seemed withdrawn some times and we were always calling his name, and trying to engage him to play and interact with us. He was fearful, terrified of things like the vacuum cleaner, people, and large trucks. Even visiting relatives would send him flying into my arms in terror. He wouldn't let people hold him or even look at him.

While he wasn't physically ill I did note a pattern of viral infections that would follow within weeks of vaccinations. By the time he was two years old, he was clearly different but we didn't know why. He was prone to constipation. He was hard to handle, fussed and didn't like food, clothing, people or going anywhere. We really had no life because we couldn't take him out much. I knew something was wrong with my boy but I didn't know what.

I stumbled upon mercury information while researching my own health issue of chronic fatigue. I discovered that amalgams were mercury fillings and that I was poisoned with 16 of them. I also learned that vaccines contained mercury and aluminum. This began my quest to find out what this meant for my children. Eventually through online forums and Andy Cutler's information I learned about hair testing and what to do about my amalgams.

My son was about 3 years old by then and used to urinate in the toilet at age two but regressed back into diapers. After his last vaccinations around age 2, I noticed his eye contact was strange. He would not look you in the eye anymore. He had this strange upward sideways glance. He was withdrawn, pale and wanted to watch the same Blue's Clue's video over and over all day. He ran around in a diaper, hated clothing and wouldn't eat food. He just wanted his bottle all the time. I had talked to the doctor numerous times about my concerns but they kept telling me he was a boy, as if that explained it. As if all boys develop that way. I knew there was more to it.

When we got his hair test results back we were devastated. He had heavy metal poisoning. It's a sad day I will never forget but I finally had an answer. We began biomedical for him first by putting him on the Feingold diet because he would turn into this violent out of control child if he ate food coloring. We took him off dairy. We started him on probiotics and he finally began to have regular stools. Then we began vitamins and prepared to chelate the lead, antimony, aluminum, arsenic, silver, tin and mercury out of him. I have to say I was nervous the first round, I was afraid that we might make him worse but the doctor didn't have any suggestions at all and I knew those metals had to come out. The doctors were not able to help us when I showed them the test results.

The first round was truly revealing for us. My son became happier than I remembered in a long time and allowed us to hug him for the first time in months. He was so different, so happy and playful that first round that we knew there definitely was something to the metals. Within five rounds he got up one morning on round and urinated in the toilet by himself. I almost fell out of bed when I heard the sound of him peeing in the toilet!

Since there was a waiting list for assessments here locally we did not get to see a developmental pediatrician until three months after chelation had begun. By this time some of my son's original symptoms were gone. Before any interventions my son scored a 118 on the ATEC and a "Definite Probable" on the Child Brain PDD Assessment. He was assessed and diagnosed with sensory integration disorder, fine motor delays and receptive language delay three months after we started biomed. He was 3 ½ years old.

Even though he had most of the symptoms of PDD they were reluctant to put it on paper because they said he could talk. And talk he did, using vocabulary beyond his years but understanding far less than he spoke. My son had scored 100 on the GADS autism screening and 104 on GARS-2 and GARS assessments at age 7, but they continued to drag their feet in case he "grew out of it".

We continued to chelate doing rounds whenever we could and eventually at age 7 they finally committed to paper the diagnosis of Asperger's Syndrome. We kept chelating because his hair testing still met rules for mercury and he continued to make gains slowly over the years in social, emotional, physical and developmental areas. He even lost his auditory processing delay.

Today he is 10 and has a few symptoms left related mainly to sensory sensitivity and some anxiety. When we stared this I did not think we would have come this far. The last assessment he had this past fall they told me they thought he was misdiagnosed because he didn't really have many features of Asperger's. Public school had plans to mainstream him for the upcoming year. However we later opted to home-school due to other issues with his school. But he isn't on Feingold anymore and can eat whatever he wants including coloring without any reaction. He's an active, inquisitive and smart young man.

While we still have some Asperger traits and sensory issues to work on, my son didn't outgrow his autism, he chelated out of it. And our story isn't over yet, not until we get a normal hair test. Today my son scores an 8 on the ATEC, and a "No PDD" on the Child Brain Assessment.

I have successfully chelated my mercury toxic daughter and myself too. We have all regained health and well being beyond my expectations from this protocol including beating my daughter's gluten allergy!

Jan Martin is the mother of two beautiful children and an active parent in the online autism community teaching parents biomedical therapies for autism. She has studied endocrine dysfunction, herbs, supplements, heavy metal toxicity, vaccines toxicology, immune function and other modalities of biomedical therapy in relation to healing from mercury poisoning.

Tressie's Story

My son was a handful. At first we thought he was just independent, stubborn, and maybe a little spoiled. He always seemed like he was in his own world, not really interested in us. Despite the fact that he talked constantly, reciting the lyrics to kids TV songs and even complete cartoon episodes, he did not have a word for Mom or Dad. He could label things when prompted, but he had no functional language. Transitions always resulted in tantrums and total meltdowns. He had night terrors, and sensory issues. He wouldn't keep his clothes on; I used safety pins and duct tape to keep him from undressing. He only wanted to eat a few preferred foods, but he would chew on anything rubber or wooden. He was hyper and did not sleep well. He would stay up late and wake up in the early morning hours wanting to play. He opened almost any door and could get around all child locks. He would try to leave the house, like an escapee waiting for any unsupervised moment to flee. He was obsessed with water, but would throw a fit if it got on his head. He did smile and laugh, but did not hug or want to be held. Even as a small baby, he never really cuddled or just relaxed in your arms.

At two and half his tantrumming had gotten worse and he still had no functional language, so I finally talked to my pediatrician. She referred us to the local school district's early education program for an evaluation. Like most parents I began searching the Internet for clues that could explain my child's delays. When I came across a checklist of symptoms, my heart sank as I answered yes to 11 out of the 12 criteria listed for Autism.

I found online biomed sites; they all recommended a gluten-free, casein-free diet. I went grocery shopping for GF/CF food the same day, desperate to help my son. The school district's report came back; he was developmentally delayed and they recommended further testing. After a couple of months on a waiting list, my son received a medical diagnosis of low-moderate functioning autism. We started taking him to a biomed doctor locally who treated yeast, and recommended zinc, B6, and fish oil. He also tested him for heavy metals and started us on a bad chelation protocol. We followed this path for a year and a half and my son did improve some, but then he refused all supplements and regressed terribly. I went back to the computer searching for something, anything I could do to help my child.

That is when I found AC chelation and it was nothing short of miraculous. From the first round we saw better eye contact, and he seemed much more engaged. Within the first twenty rounds he was answering us from the other room. Before AC he would ignore you even if you called him repeatedly right by his head. He was asking questions, using "W" words, even making jokes. At five years of age, my never sick son got the sniffles, then a minor cold. I'd never been so happy to see someone ill before. I lived, breathed, ate, and slept at my computer spending hours researching and listening to advice from other parents. It was grueling, but I was learning how to get my child back, and it was working.

We had him reassessed for ASD and after a year and a half of AC chelation, his diagnosis was lightened to PDD-NOS. We kept chelating and supplementing and dieting. Another year passed and the following summer he was reassessed. This time he received no diagnosis at all. They read his history and told me they knew he had ASD, but they could not find it. It simply didn't show up on any of the tests. He entered Kindergarten at 6 years old with no aid or classroom supports, and NO DIAGNOSIS! They said the only support he tested for was speech, to help him better pronounce the letter "L". It was unbelievable! I knew he had come so far from where we started, but even I was surprised by this news. He did wonderfully. The principal thought he was very bright and recommended him for IQ testing. He scored as moderately gifted and is now in a program for highly intelligent children.

What is more exciting to me are his social activities. He spends most of his time outside playing with his younger brother and the other neighborhood boys. There are 5 or 6 of them and he gets along with all of them (most of the time, although there have been a disagreement or two, WOW so typical.) They regularly ring our doorbell and ask for him to come out and play. We still have a few minor issues. He has larger vocabulary than most boys his age, and sometimes uses an odd vocal inflection. He sometimes has a slightly irregular posture, but that is all I can find to distinguish him from his peers. He no longer needs special diets. He can eat cake and ice cream, pizza, candy, red slushies, and chocolate without any change in behavior. He doesn't need the barrage of anti-fungals and probiotics, B6, B12, fatty acids, vitamin A, Epsom salts baths, and a slew of other things we used daily just to help him function and think clearly. He is only taking a few support supplements for general health and wellness. We are still belting out the rounds hoping to get rid of the few, tiny issues we have left. Of course now everyone in the house is chelating, even Dad. The entire family is seeing amazing health benefits. We have been truly blessed with this knowledge and I want to share it with the world.

Tressie Taylor is the mother of 6 wonderful children and an active parent advocate and coach for natural biomedical therapies to treat autism. She is currently training to be an herbalist and has formally studied nutrition, herbal medicine and natural diets in addition to supplements.

Bibliography

Adams, James B., Matthew Baral, Elizabeth Geis, Jessica Mitchell, Julie Ingram, Andrea Hensley, Irene Zappia, Sanford Newmark, Eva Gehn, Robert A. Rubin, Ken Mitchell, Jeff Bradstreet, and Jane El-Dahr. "Safety and Efficacy of Oral DMSA Therapy for Children with Autism Spectrum Disorders: Part A - Medical Results." *BMC Clinical Pharmacology* 9.1 2009):16. Print. <http://www.ncbi.nlm.nih.gov/pubmed/19852789>

"Adrenal Glands". *Tuberose.com Natural Healing Products and Information for Transformation.* Web. 27 Aug. 2011. <http://tuberose.com>

Al-Gadani, Y., A. El-Ansary, O. Attas, and L. Al-Ayadhi. "Metabolic Biomarkers Related to Oxidative Stress and Antioxidant Status in Saudi Autistic Children." *Clinical Biochemistry* 42.10-11 (2009): 1032-040. Print. <http://www.ncbi.nlm.nih.gov/pubmed/19306862>

"Atherosclerosis, Prostate Health, Hormones, Diabetes, and More Health Concerns – Life Extension". *Highest Quality Vitamins and Supplements-Life Extension.* 1995-2011. Web. 31 Aug. 2011. <http://www.lef.org/protocols/>

Biewenga, G., G. Haenen, and A. Bast. "The Pharmacology of the Antioxidant Lipoic Acid." *General Pharmacology: The Vascular System* 29.3 (1997): 315-31. Print. <http://www.ncbi.nlm.nih.gov/pubmed/9378235>.

Bowthorpe, Janie A. *Stop the Thyroid Madness: a Patient Revolution against Decades of Inferior Thyroid Treatment.* Florence, CO: Laughing Grape Pub., 2008. Print. <http://www.laughinggrapepublishing.com/all-about-the-book/>

Britton, S. W., and H. Silvette. "Further Experiments On Corticoadrenal Extract: Its Efficacy By Mouth." *Science* 74 (1931):440-41. <http://www.ncbi.nlm.nih.gov/pubmed/17793908>

Chauhan, A., and V. Chauhan. "Oxidative Stress in Autism."
Pathophysiology 13.3 (2006): 171-81.
Print.<http://69.164.208.4/files/OXIDATIVE%20STRESS%20IN%20
AUTISM.pdf>.

Connett, P. H., James S. Beck, and H. S. Micklem. *The Case against
Fluoride: How Hazardous Waste Ended up in Our Drinking Water and the Bad
Science and Powerful Politics That Keep It There.* White River Junction, VT:
Chelsea Green Pub., 2010. Print
<http://www.fluorideresearch.org/433/files/FJ2010_v43_n3_p170-
173.pdf>

Clark, Hulda Regehr. *The Cure for All Diseases.* Chula Vista, CA: New
Century, 2006. Print. ISBN978-1890035013

Crook, William G. *The Yeast Connection: a Medical Breakthrough.* New York:
Vintage, 1986. Print. ISBN978-0394747002

Cutler, Andrew Hall. *Amalgam Illness: Diagnosis and Treatment.* Irvine, CA.:
Andrew Hall Cutler, 1999. Print. ISBN 0967616808
<http://www.noamalgam.com/>

Hair Test Interpretation: Finding Hidden Toxicities. Sammamish, Wash:
Andrew Hall Cutler, 2004. Print. ISBN 0967616816
<http://www.noamalgam.com/hairtestbook.html>

Cutler Protocol – "OnibasuWiki." *Onibasu.com:* Web. 27 Aug. 2011.
<http://onibasu.com/wiki/Cutler_protocol>.

Cysteine Status – "OnibasuWiki" *Onibasu.com:* Web. 27 Aug. 2011.
<http://onibasu.com/wiki/Cysteine_status>.

Davis, Adelle. *Let's Get Well.* New York: Harcourt, Brace & World, 1965.
Print ISBN978-0451154637

DL-α±-Lipoic Acid • Thioctic Acid (CAS 1077-28-7) || Cayman
Chemical." *Home || Cayman Chemical.* 2011. Web. 27 Aug. 2011.

<http://www.caymanchem.com/app/template/Product.vm/catalog/100 05728>.

Durrant-Peatfield, Barry. *The Great Thyroid Scandal and How to Survive It.* London: Barons Down, 2002. Print. ISBN978-0954420307

Enzymes & Viruses. EnzymeStuff Site – "Everything about Digestive Enzymes". Web. 27 Aug. 2011 <http://enzymestuff.com/conditionviruses.htm>.

Environmental Working Group" Environmental Working Group, 2007. Web. 25 Aug. 2011 http://www.ewg.org/tap-water/home

Fallon, Sally, Mary G. Enig, Kim Murray, and Marion Dearth. *Nourishing Traditions: the Cookbook That Challenges Politically Correct Nutrition and the Diet Dictocrats.* Washington, DC: NewTrends Pub., 2001. Print. ISBN 0967089735

Feingold, Ben F. *Why Your Child Is Hyperactive.* New York: Random House, 1996. Print ISBN978-0394734262.

"Feingold Diet Program for ADHD, The". Web. 27 Aug. 2011. <http://feingold.org>.

"Fish Women Should Avoid | Environmental Working Group." Web. 25 Aug. 2011.<http://ewg.org/safefishlist>.

GAPS Diet. Web. 27 Aug. 2011. <http://gapsdiet.com>.

Gates, Donna. *The Body Ecology Diet, Healthy Diets -BodyEcology.com.* Web. 27 Aug. 2011. http://bodyecology.com>.

Gluten Free. Web. 27 Aug. 2011. http://glutenfree.com

Haas, Elson M., and Buck Levin. *Staying Healthy with Nutrition: the Complete Guide to Diet and Nutritional Medicine.* Berkeley: Celestial Arts, 2006. Print. ISBN978-0890874813.

How to Use a Rotation Diet; Food-Allergy.org. *How to Survive with Multiple Food Allergies and Eventually Thrive Again.* Web. 27 Aug. 2011. <http://food-allergy.org/rotation.html>.

"How We Get Parasites." Humaworm.com. n.p., 2010-2011. Web. 27 Aug. 2011. <http://humaworm.com>.

Huggins, Hal A. *It's All in Your Head: the Link between Mercury Amalgams and Illness.* Garden City Park, NY: Avery Pub Group. 1993. Print. ISBN978-0895295507

IAOMT. "The Toxic Effects of Dental Amalgam". August 2011 <http://www.iaomt.org/articles/files/files342/IAOMT%20Fact%20Sheet.pdf>.

"Mercury Free Dentistry, Mercury Safe Dentists, Fluoride Free Dentists" Web. 27 Aug. http://www.iaomt.org/patients/search.aspx>.

Jefferies, William McK. *Safe Uses of Cortisol.* Springfield, IL: Charles C. Thomas, 2004. Print. ISBN978-0398066215.

Kozma, Láaszló, Lajos Papp, Éva Varga, and Szabolcs Gomba. "Accumulation of Hg(II) Ions in Mouse Adrenal Gland." *Pathology & Oncology Research* 2.1-2 (1996): 52-55. Print <http://www.ncbi.nlm.nih.gov/pubmed/11173584>

Matthews, Julie. *Nourishing Hope: Nutrition Intervention for Autism Spectrum Disorders.*[S.l.]: Nourishing Hope, 2007. Print ISBN978-0981655802 <http://www.noamalgam.com/nourishinghope.html>

"Metabolic Therapy Overview." Dr.Rind. n.d. Web. 27 Aug. 2011. http://www.drrind.com/therapies/metabolic-therapy

Miller, Neil Z. "Aluminum in Vaccines: A Neurological Gamble." (2009). Web. 25 Aug. 2011. <http://thinktwice.com/aluminum.pdf>.

Murray, Michael T., *Encyclopedia of Nutritional Supplements: the Essential Guide for Improving Your Health Naturally.* Rocklin, CA: Prima Pub., 1996. Print. ISBN978-0761504108.

Murray, Michael T., and Joseph E. Pizzorno. *Encyclopedia of Natural Medicine*. Rocklin, CA: Prima Pub., 1998. Print ISBN978-0761511571

"NIH Mercury-Free Campaign." *National Institute of Health*. n.p. Web. 27 Aug. 2011 <http://orf.od.nih.gov/Environmental+Protection/Mercury+Free/>.

Ou, P. "Thioctic (lipoic) Acid: a Therapeutic Metal-chelating Antioxidant?" *Biochemical Pharmacology* 50.1 (1995): 123-26. Print. <http://www.ncbi.nlm.nih.gov/pubmed/7605337>

Price, Weston A. *Nutrition and Physical Degeneration*. La Mesa, CA: Price-Pottenger Nutrition Foundation, 2008. Print. ISBN978-0879838164.

Rankin, RN, CRNA, Sym C. "Anesthesia & the Autistic Child." *The Autism File* (2009). Web. 27 Aug. 2011. <http://www.autismone.org/content/anesthesia-autistic-child-sym-c-rankin-rn-crna>.

"RecoveryFromAutism : Recovery From Autism." *Yahoo! Groups : Directory : Health & Wellness*. Parent reports. Mar. 2009. Web. 27 Aug. 2011. <http://health.groups.yahoo.com/group/RecoveryFromAutism/>.

Report of a Joint FAO/WHO Expert Consultation. "Health and Nutritional Properties of Probiotics in." *Food and Agriculture Organization*. World Health Organization, Oct. 2001. Web. 27 Aug. 2011. <http://www.who.int/foodsafety/publications/fs_management/en/probiotics.pdf>.

Rooney, James K. Corrigendum to "The Role of Thiols, Dithiols, Nutritional Factors and Interacting Ligands in the Toxicology of Mercury" [Toxicology 234 (2007) 145–156]. *Toxicology* 238.2-3 (2007): 216. Print. <http://www.sciencedirect.com/science/article/pii/S0300483X07004350>

SafeMinds. "Autism Mercury Thimerosal". Web. 25 Aug. 2011.
<http://safeminds.org/mercury/history.html>.

Scdiet.org - SCD Web Library - Natural Remission of Crohn's, Colitis, IBD. Web.
27 Aug. 2011. <http://scdiet.org>.

"Scientific Review of Vaccine Safety Datalink Information" June 7-8
2000, Simpsonwood Retreat Center, Norcross, Georgia
<http://www.nationalautismassociation.org/pdf/simpsonwood.pdf>

Shaw, William, and Bernard Rimland. *Biological Treatments for Autism and
PDD.* Lenexa, Kan.: W. Shaw, 2002. Print. ISBN978-0966123814.
<http://www.noamalgam.com/biologicaltreatments.html>

Strambi, Mirella, Mariangela Longini, Joseph Hayek, Silvia Berni,
Francesca Macucci, Elisa Scalacci, and Piero Vezzosi. "Magnesium
Profile in Autism." *Biological Trace Element Research* 109.2 (2006): 097-104.
Print. <http://www.ncbi.nlm.nih.gov/pubmed/16443999>

Studies Have Documented That Mercury Causes Hypothyroidism
(50,84,390), damage of Thyroid RNA (458), Autoimmune Thyroiditis (36
"Florida League of Conservation Voters Education Fund". Web. 27 Aug. 2011.
<http://flcv.com/ASDendo.html>.

Thyroid Antibodies: The Test *"Lab Tests Online: Welcome!"* Web. 27 Aug.
2011. <http://labtestsonline.org/understanding/analytes/thyroid-
antibodies/tab/test>.

"Vaccines are not mercury free" by Health Advocacy in the Public
Interest (HAPI), Dawn Winkler, August, 12, 2004
<http://www.medkb.com/Uwe/Forum.aspx/alternative/6380/Vaccines
-Are-Not-Mercury-Free>.

Weston A. Price Foundation, The-Weston A Price Foundation. Web. 27 Aug.
2011. http://westonaprice.org

United States. Environmental Protection Agency. "What You Need to
Know about Mercury in Fish and Shellfish". EPA, 2004. Web.25

Aug.2011.
<http://water.epa.gov/scitech/swguidance/fishshellfish/outreach/advic
e_index.cfm>

Wilson, James L. *Adrenal Fatigue: the 21st Century Stress Syndrome.* Petaluma,
CA: Smart Publications, 2007. Print. ISBN9781890572150

CPSIA information can be obtained
at www.ICGtesting.com
Printed in the USA
FFOW01n1048180318
45700875-46541FF